Allergy, Asthma, and Immunology

Editor

GABRIEL ORTIZ

PHYSICIAN ASSISTANT CLINICS

www.physicianassistant.theclinics.com

Consulting Editors
KIM ZUBER
JANE S. DAVIS

October 2023 • Volume 8 • Number 4

ELSEVIER

1600 John F. Kennedy Boulevard • Suite 1800 • Philadelphia, Pennsylvania, 19103-2899

http://www.theclinics.com

PHYSICIAN ASSISTANT CLINICS Volume 8, Number 4
October 2023 ISSN 2405-7991, ISBN-13: 978-0-323-93841-9

Editor: Taylor Hayes
Developmental Editor: Saswoti Nath

Physician Assistant Clinics (ISSN: 2405–7991) is published quarterly by Elsevier Inc., 360 Park Avenue South, New York, NY 10010-1710. Months of issue are January, April, July, and October. Periodicals postage paid at New York, NY and additional mailing offices. Subscription prices are $150.00 per year (US individuals), $305.00 (US institutions), $100.00 (US students), $150.00 (Canadian individuals), $320.00 (Canadian institutions), $100.00 (Canadian students), $150.00 (international individuals), $320.00 (international institutions), and $100.00 (international students). Foreign air speed delivery is included in all *Clinics* subscription prices. All prices are subject to change without notice. POSTMASTER: Send address changes to *Physician Assistant Clinics*, Elsevier Periodicals Customer Service, 11830 Westline Industrial Drive, St. Louis, MO 63146. Customer Service Health Sciences Division, Subscription Customer Service, 3251 Riverport Lane, Maryland Heights, MO 63043. **Customer Service: 1-800-654-2452 (U.S. and Canada); 314-447-8871 (outside U.S. and Canada). Fax: 314-447-8029. E-mail: journalscustomerservice-usa@elsevier.com (for print support); journalsonlinesupport-usa@elsevier.com (for online support).**

Reprints. For copies of 100 or more, of articles in this publication, please contact the Commercial Reprints Department, Elsevier Inc., 360 Park Avenue South, New York, NY 10010-1710. Tel. 212-633-3874; Fax: 212-633-3820; E-mail: reprints@elsevier.com.

Physician Assistant Clinics is covered in *EMBASE/Excerpta Medica and ESCI.*

PROGRAM OBJECTIVE
The goal of the *Physician Assistant Clinics* is to keep practicing physician assistants up to date with current clinical practice by providing timely articles reviewing the state of the art in patient care.

TARGET AUDIENCE
Physician Assistants and other healthcare professionals

LEARNING OBJECTIVES
Upon completion of this activity, participants will be able to:
1. Review the prevalence of food allergies as a growing global health concern and a hot topic in the allergy and asthma field.
2. Discuss the clinical manifestations and variety of respiratory symptoms associated with asthma.
3. Recognize it is crucial to understand the significance of proper screening and referrals for patients with atopic diseases due to the risk of comorbid mental health problems.

ACCREDITATION
The Elsevier Office of Continuing Medical Education (EOCME) is accredited by the Accreditation Council for Continuing Medical Education (ACCME) to provide continuing medical education for physicians.

The EOCME designates this journal-based CME activity for a maximum of 13 *AMA PRA Category 1 Credit*(s)™. Physicians should claim only the credit commensurate with the extent of their participation in the activity.

All other health care professionals requesting continuing education credit for this enduring material will be issued a certificate of participation.

DISCLOSURE OF CONFLICTS OF INTEREST
The EOCME assesses conflict of interest with its instructors, faculty, planners, and other individuals who are in a position to control the content of CME activities. All relevant conflicts of interest that are identified are thoroughly vetted by EOCME for fair balance, scientific objectivity, and patient care recommendations. EOCME is committed to providing its learners with CME activities that promote improvements or quality in healthcare and not a specific proprietary business or a commercial interest.

The planning committee, staff, authors, and editors listed below have identified no financial relationships or relationships to products or devices they or their spouse/life partner have with commercial interest related to the content of this CME activity:
Brian Bizik, PA-C; Tina L.R. Dominguez, PA-C, MMS; Keri Holyoak, MPH, MSHS, PA-C; Kothainayaki Kulanthaivelu, BCA, MBA; Michelle Littlejohn; David Mangold, BS, MHS, PA-C; Gabriel R. Ortiz, MPAS, PA-C, DFAAPA; Kimberly Poarch, MPAS, PA-C; William D. Sanders, DMS, PA-C; Nicole Soucy, MPAS PA-C; Jennifer Watson, MN, FNP-C

The planning committee, staff, authors, and editors listed below have identified financial relationships or relationships to products or devices they or their spouse/life partner have with commercial interest related to the content of this CME activity:
Tara Bruner, MHS, PA-C, DFAAPA: Employee: Thermo Fisher Scientific

Scott Duhaime, MPAS, PA-C: Employee: Thermo Fisher Scientific

Gary Falcetano, PA-C, AE-C: Employee: Thermo Fisher Scientific

Tamara Hubbard, MA, LCPC: Honoraria: Novartis, Regeneron, Thermo Fisher Scientific

Amanda Michaud, DMSc, PA-C, AE-C: Honoraria: Novartis, Regeneron, Thermo Fisher Scientific

UNAPPROVED/OFF-LABEL USE DISCLOSURE
The EOCME requires CME faculty to disclose to the participants:
1. When products or procedures being discussed are off-label, unlabelled, experimental, and/or investigational (not US Food and Drug Administration [FDA] approved); and
2. Any limitations on the information presented, such as data that are preliminary or that represent ongoing research, interim analyses, and/or unsupported opinions. Faculty may discuss information about pharmaceutical agents that is outside of FDA-approved labelling. This information is intended solely for CME and is not intended to promote off-label use of these medications. If you have any questions, contact the medical affairs department of the manufacturer for the most recent prescribing information.

TO ENROLL

The CME program is available to all *Physician Assistant Clinics* subscribers at no additional fee. To subscribe to the *Physician Assistant Clinics*, call customer service at 1-800-654-2452 or sign up online at www.physicianassistant.theclinics.com. The CME program is available to subscribers for an additional annual fee of USD 149.00.

METHOD OF PARTICIPATION

In order to claim credit, participants must complete the following:
1. Complete enrolment as indicated above
2. Read the activity
3. Complete the CME Test and Evaluation. Participants must achieve a score of 70% on the test. All CME Tests and Evaluations must be completed online

CME INQUIRIES/SPECIAL NEEDS

For all CME inquiries or special needs, please contact elsevierCME@elsevier.com.

Contributors

CONSULTING EDITORS

KIM ZUBER, PA-C, MS
American Academy of Nephrology PAs, St Petersburg, Florida

JANE S. DAVIS, CRNP, DNP
Division of Nephrology, The University of Alabama at Birmingham, Birmingham, Alabama

EDITOR

GABRIEL ORTIZ, MPAS, PA-C, DFAAPA
BS Microbiology, BS Medical Technology, BS Physician Assistant Studies, MPAS Pediatric Pulmonary Medicine, Executive Clinical Educator, Thermo Fisher Scientific, Portage, Michigan

AUTHORS

BRAIN BIZIK, MS, PA-C
Clinical Supervisor, Asthma and COPD Care Coordinator, Terry Reilly, Health Centers, Nampa, Idaho

TARA BRUNER, MHS, PA-C, DFAAPA
Senior Clinical Educator, ImmunoDiagnostics, Thermo Fisher Scientific, Portage, Michigan

TINA L.R. DOMINGUEZ, PA-C, MMS
East Bay Clinical Director, Latitude Food Allergy Care, San Ramon, California; Speaker and Consultant, Aimmune Therapeutics, Sean N. Parker Center for Allergy & Asthma Research

SCOTT DUHAIME, MPAS, PA-C
Executive Clinical Educator, ImmunoDiagnostics, Thermo Fisher Scientific, Portage, Michigan

GARY FALCETANO, PA-C, AE-C
Thermo Fisher Scientific, Portage, Michigan

KERI HOLYOAK, MPH, MSHS, PA-C
The Dermatology Center of Salt Lake, Midvale, Utah

TAMARA HUBBARD, MA, LCPC
Private practice, LCPC, LLC, Long Grove, Illinois

DAVID MANGOLD, BS, MHS, PA-C
Allergy & Asthma Center, PC, Kalispell, Montana

AMANDA MICHAUD, DMSC, PA-C, AE-C
Physician Assistant, Allergy and Immunology Family Allergy and Asthma Consultants, Dallas, Texas

KIMBERLY POARCH, MPAS, PA-C
Allergy and Asthma Specialists, Dallas, Texas

WILLIAM D. SANDERS, DMS, PA-C
Member of ACAAI (American College of Allergy, Asthma, and Immunology), Immediate Past President of APA-AAI, Allergy Specialty Care, Lake City, Florida

NICOLE SOUCY, MPAS, PA-C
Association of Physician Assistants in Allergy, Asthma, and Immunology, Board of Directors, Dallas, Texas

JENNIFER WATSON, MN, FNP-C
Asthma & Allergy of Idaho, Coeur d'Alene, Idaho

Contents

> This article offers a concise overview of the history and understanding of allergic-mediated conditions including the heterogenous condition of asthma. Beginning with early descriptions of asthma and allergic rhinitis, Falcetano describes the connection between allergy and asthma and how our knowledge of these conditions has evolved throughout history. The progression of allergy diagnostic testing from crude skin testing in the late nineteenth century through the molecular diagnostics of the 21 first century are described in detail. *Allergy and Asthma from the Beginning* concludes with a look at the sometimes prescient and insightful, sometimes dangerous therapies of early asthma and allergy treatment and their progression to modern day targeted biologic interventions.

> The immune system is a complex network of cells, chemicals, and processes that protect the body from foreign antigens. Primary immunodeficiencies are inherited disorders of immune dysregulation that can result in recurrent and severe infections, autoimmune disease, increased inflammation, and malignancies. Clinicians must be aware of the warning signs of primary immunodeficiencies and when to refer patients to clinical immunologists for proper evaluation of recurrent infections. This review serves as a basic primer on immunology, and discusses the signs and symptoms of immunodeficiency. There is also a focus on the screening, diagnosis, and basic management of immunodeficiency.

> Allergic rhinitis is an IgE-mediated sensitivity to aeroallergens that impacts millions of individuals worldwide. Previously believed to be a bothersome "disease of the nose," its impact on the entire respiratory system has become better understood in recent years. Uncontrolled allergic rhinitis can lead to the development of asthma. In individuals with comorbid asthma,

imbalances in the control of allergic rhinitis can lead to exacerbations of asthma. Understanding the epidemiological factors, symptoms, diagnosis, and treatments available for allergic rhinitis is key to maintaining a healthy airway and can improve patient outcomes.

Asthma is characterized by variable respiratory symptoms and airflow limitation and is a consequence of complex genetic and environmental interactions. The goal of treatment is to achieve and maintain symptom control while allowing patients to live normal lives with limited exacerbations. This article will review the similarities and differences between the Global Initiative for Asthma report guidelines and the National Asthma Education and Prevention Program.

Asthma is a common respiratory disease that affects children, and it is characterized by chronic inflammation and hyperreactivity in the airway. Utilization of risk prediction tools, recognition of symptoms, accurate diagnosis, and initiation of proper treatment in a timely manner can prevent significant morbidity and severity of symptoms. Multiple avenues of treatment include effective trigger avoidance measures, proper pharmacologic therapy, allergen immunotherapy in appropriate patients, and close medical follow-up; implementation of these treatment modalities will benefit pediatric patients with asthma.

Allergy diagnostics can have an important role in managing patient allergies. Knowledge is power with clinical assessment of the patient, whole allergen testing, and the addition of in vitro component allergen testing. Clinicians can make a more informed decision by increasing test sensitivity and analytical specificity with this component diagnostics for food allergy, pet allergy, Hymenoptera allergy, and alpha-Gal.

Oral food challenges are the gold standard test that can distinguish immunoglobulin (Ig)E-mediated from non-IgE-mediated food allergies. Although widely used in research, oral food challenges are underused in clinical practice for a variety of reasons. Determining when, how, and why to conduct an oral food challenge can seem like a daunting task. Serum IgE, skin prick testing, and clinical history can assist in determining the outcome of an oral food challenge, but it cannot guarantee that the patient will successfully pass an oral food challenge. Yet, the impact of an oral food challenge for some is immeasurable.

and latex. The clinical presentation can vary greatly which can make diagnosis difficult. Understanding of the variable pathophysiology, common triggers, symptoms, and treatment of anaphylaxis is essential for patient outcomes. Epinephrine is always the first-line treatment in anaphylaxis. Patients who are at risk for or who have experienced anaphylaxis should be evaluated by an allergist, have access to injectable epinephrine, and have an outlined emergency care plan for future episodes.

Discussions of Asthma COPD Overlap (ACO), the condition of having asthma and COPD in the same individual, began in the early 1960s. Since that time, researchers and clinicians have debated what to call the overlap and whether it is an extension of asthma and/or COPD or a separate disease altogether. None of the many helpful biomarkers that researchers have discovered are pathognomonic, however. That fact aside, it is important for clinicians to diagnose these patients properly because studies have shown they have exacerbations that lead to increased hospital admission rates. As recently as 2022, clinicians were prescribing treatments normally used for asthma and patients with COPD to assess their efficacy in treating patients who have ACO.

PHYSICIAN ASSISTANT CLINICS

SERIES OF RELATED INTEREST

Primary Care: Clinics in Office Practice
https://www.primarycare.theclinics.com/
Immunology & Allergy Clinics
https://www.immunology.theclinics.com/

THE CLINICS ARE AVAILABLE ONLINE!
Access your subscription at:
www.theclinics.com

Foreword
Allergy, Asthma, and Immunology

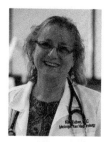 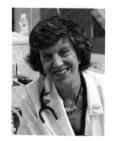

Kim Zuber, PA-C, MS   Jane S. Davis, CRNP, DNP
Consulting Editors

It began with a sneeze or maybe a rash or even a wheeze. But somewhere, long ago, there was a realization that often elements in the environment can cause unpleasant reactions. And the study of allergy, asthma, and immunology was born.

In 1999, the American Academy of Physician Associates formally recognized the Association of Allergy, Asthma and Immunology PAs. One of their main goals is education, and so we present allergy, asthma, and immunology by and from our colleague experts for an issue of *Physician Assistant Clinics*. Gabriel Ortiz has assembled a group of experts from across the country to give us the background on what these conditions are, where they originate, how they present, and details on how best to manage them.

Included is the conflict between the United States and the rest of the world on management of asthma, a virtual war without weapons but with very strong opinions and supportive research instead. Ever wondered how to describe a skin condition or sort asthma from COPD? These expert authors have you covered.

While a rash is not usually an emergency, extreme shortness of breath is. From food allergies to environmental triggers to man-made products, almost any product can provoke a response in some people.

Physician Assist Clin 8 (2023) xiii–xiv
https://doi.org/10.1016/j.cpha.2023.07.003
2405-7991/23/© 2023 Published by Elsevier Inc.

These are just a few highlights of what awaits in the interesting and educational issue of *Physician Assistant Clinics*. We hope you enjoy and benefit from the insight and information in this issue. I know it will be a part of our resource libraries for years to come.

Kim Zuber, PA-C, MS
American Academy of Nephrology PAs
131 31st Avenue North
St Petersburg, FL 33704, USA

Jane S. Davis, CRNP, DNP
Division of Nephrology
University of Alabama at Birmingham
3605 Oakdale Road
Birmingham, AL 35223, USA

E-mail addresses:
zuberkim@yahoo.com (K. Zuber)
jsdavis@uabmc.edu (J.S. Davis)

Preface

Overview of the Essential Knowledge for Clinical Practice in Allergy and Immunology

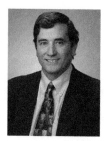

Gabriel Ortiz, MPAS, PA-C, DFAAPA
Editor

This issue on Allergy and Immunology is a timely issue. As the current trend of allergic disease is rising, this issue will be beneficial to any health care provider (HCP). Physician assistants in the allergy/immunology field are begining to increase year after year as we see fewer and fewer allergist in this medical field. There has been an increase in allergic disease in the last several years. This will be a great reference for allergic disease because the field of allergy is not very well studied in PA school.

When we discuss allergic diseases, we should keep in mind what is called the "Atopic March."[1] A group of seemingly unrelated diseases that can begin with eczema or more appropriately atopic dermatitis then can proceed to food allergy and then to allergic rhinitis and culmination of these allergic diseases with allergic asthma. All these more common allergic diseases are discussed in this issue.

In the United States, allergic diseases, such as asthma, allergic rhinitis (hay fever), eczema (atopic dermatitis), and food allergy, are common for all age groups. Allergic diseases are a common cause of illness with more than 50 million Americans suffering from allergies each year. More than 24 million people in the United States suffer from asthma, including more than 6 million children.[2]

In the United States, allergies are listed as the sixth leading cause of chronic illness.[2] Food allergies have increased significantly in children from 3.4% in 1997–1999 to 5.1% in 2009–2011.[3] Food allergies affect about 32 million people in the United States,[4,5] affecting about 5.6 million children (7.6%)[5] and about 26 million adults (10.8%).[4]

Physician Assist Clin 8 (2023) xv–xvii
https://doi.org/10.1016/j.cpha.2023.07.002
2405-7991/23/© 2023 Published by Elsevier Inc.

Over the past 20 years, food allergy has been increasing among US children with the greatest increase seen in black children.[5]

Nine foods are responsible for over 90% of food allergies, with milk the most common food allergen in children, followed by egg and peanut,[6] and for adults, shellfish is the most common allergen, followed by peanut and tree nuts.[6] In the United States, sesame is a rising food allergy that has an estimated impact on 1 million people.[7] In 2021, sesame was declared a major allergen and added to the previous list of the eight most common foods.

The LEAP (Learning Early About Peanut Allergy) Study published in 2012 by Du Toit and colleagues[8] and subsequent articles have given the allergy community enough clinical information to now recommend early introduction of peanut protein into the infant's diet.[9] This is an advancement that has been made in the field of allergy research.

We have seen a great many clinical trials and new FDA-approved medications in the allergy field in the last 30 years. There have been great discoveries that have shown inflammation plays a major role in the allergic cascade. This recent clinical research has led to the FDA approval of several new biologic agents for the treatment of several allergic diseases.

There have also been several new allergy diagnostic tests approved to help in the field of allergy. These new diagnostic tests allow the HCP to make a more precise diagnosis. The field of allergy has been more accepting of the therapeutic approach to use Oral Immunotherapy, much like we use subcutaneous immunotherapy (allergy shots).

We begin this issue with an overview by Falcetano on the history of allergic disease and some early clinical information that has led to much of our early understanding of allergic disease. This issue adds to the basic immunology and primary immunodeficiencies by Michaud and Watson. Soucy discusses allergic rhinitis and asthma in the adult population, including the important concept of the united airway.

Many of the more recent publications on asthma have been regarding the asthma guidelines, and Bizik discusses the differences between the National Institutes of Health guidelines and the Global Initiative of Asthma guidelines. There has been significant research in the pediatric allergy field, and Watson and Poarch review the latest updates for clinical pediatric allergy and asthma. Allergy diagnostics has improved drastically in the last several years, and Bruner and Duhaime review these newer diagnostic tests that will help any HCP make a more precise diagnosis for better patient management.

Dominquez discusses the current thoughts on pediatric food allergy, including oral food challenges. The Psychosocial aspects of allergy and asthma are detailed by Hubbard and Michaud. There are several important procedures in the allergy practice that are discussed by Mangold. As atopic dermatitis plays a major role in the allergic field, Holyoak explains atopic dermatitis and differentiates several masqueraders of atopic dermatitis. Michaud and Soucy elaborate on Anaphylaxis with several different triggers. This issue will conclude with a timely article on Asthma-COPD overlap by Sanders.

This issue on Allergy and Immunology is an extensive basic knowledge primer for any HCP interested in the Allergy/Immunology field. This issue covers a wide range of topics that should be very familiar to any HCP treating patients with these allergic diseases. Since more Physician Assistants are entering the field of allergy, this reference will be a welcome addition.

Gabriel Ortiz, MPAS, PA-C, DFAAPA
Thermo Fisher Scientific
4169 Commercial Avenue
Portage, MI 49002, USA

E-mail address:
aapaaai99@yahoo.com

REFERENCES

1. Tsuge M, Ikeda M, Matsumoto N, et al. Current insights into atopic march. Children (Basel) 2021;8(11):1067.
2. American College of Allergy, Asthma, and Immunology. (2018). Allergy facts. Available at: https://acaai.org/news/facts-statistics/allergies. Accessed June 1, 2022.
3. Available at: https://www.cdc.gov/nchs/data/databriefs/db121.pdf. Accessed June 1, 2022.
4. Gupta RS, Warren CM, Smith BM, et al. Prevalence and severity of food allergies among US adults. JAMA Network Open 2019;2(1):e185630. https://doi.org/10.1001/jamanetworkopen.2018.5630.
5. Gupta RS, Warren CM, Smith BM, et al. The public health impact of parent-reported childhood food allergies in the United States. Pediatrics 2018;142(6). https://doi.org/10.1542/peds.2018-1235.
6. Iweala OI, Choudhary SK, Commins SP. Food allergy. Curr Gastroenterol Rep 2018;20(5):17. https://doi.org/10.1007/s11894-018-0624-y.
7. Warren CM, Chadha AS, Sicherer SH, et al. Prevalence and severity of sesame allergy in the United States. JAMA Network Open 2019;2(8):e199144. https://doi.org/10.1001/jamanetworkopen.2019.9144.
8. Du Toit G, Roberts G, Sayre PH, et al, Learning Early About Peanut Allergy (LEAP) Study Team. Identifying infants at high risk of peanut allergy: the Learning Early About Peanut Allergy (LEAP) screening study. J Allergy Clin Immunol 2013; 131(1):135–43.
9. Chang A, Cabana MD, LaFlam TN, et al. Early peanut introduction and testing: a framework for general pediatrician beliefs and practices. Pediatr Allergy Immunol Pulmonol 2021;34(2):53–9.

Allergy and Asthma from the Beginning

Gary Falcetano, PA-C, AE-C

KEYWORDS

- Allergy • Asthma • Allergen • Respiratory disease • Food allergy
- Allergen immunotherapy • Bronchodilator • Antihistamine

KEY POINTS

- Although the understanding of asthma and allergy has broadened over time, early observations of their strong association have remained true.
- Environmental effects on both allergy and asthma were observed early and have remained key drivers of these conditions today.
- As diagnostics and therapeutics have evolved, a more personalized understanding of each patient's disease has allowed for better targeted lifestyle modifications and therapeutic interventions.

Allergic diseases including asthma, which is a heterogenous disease predominately mediated by allergy, have been described in writings of various cultures throughout the world for thousands of years. Numerous descriptions using terms such as "asthma," "eczema" and "idiosyncrasy" can be found in ancient writings and remain part of our current medical lexicon.[1]

Early Descriptions of Asthma

The term "asthma" has its origins from the Greek verb "aazein" meaning to exhale with open mouth, to pant. It's first use in a medical context is found in the *Corpus Hippocraticum* where Hippocrates (460–377 BCE) described the constellation of symptoms consistent with the actual disease.[2]

The English physician Henry Hyde Salter (1823–1871) later described asthma and the associated physiologic mechanisms in his publication from 1860, *On asthma its pathology and treatment*. Salter defined asthma as "paroxysmal dyspnoea of a peculiar character with intervals of healthy respiration between attacks" what we now refer to as reversibility. He also quite remarkably detailed cellular illustrations of the airways in patients with asthma depicting what are now known to be eosinophils and mast cells and also described his concept of this disease that was exacerbated by narrowing of the airways due to smooth muscle contraction. Salter also was aware of the

Thermo Fisher Scientific, 4169 Commercial Avenue, Portage, MI 49002, USA
E-mail address: gary.falcetano@thermofisher.com

Physician Assist Clin 8 (2023) 613–620
https://doi.org/10.1016/j.cpha.2023.06.001
2405-7991/23/

apparent effects of heredity and "idiosyncrasies" emanating from horses, cats, and other animals, today we understand as some of the environmental allergens that effect allergic asthma. Henry Salter who suffered with asthma himself, most likely based the content of his writings on his own personal experience as well as the hundreds of cases he attended in his medical practice. Interestingly, he also described hot strong black coffee as a treatment for these muscle contractions (spasms.) Coffee as we are now aware, contains caffeine, a drug with similar although less potent, broncho-dilatory properties to theophylline.[3]

Seasonal Allergic Rhinitis–Hay Fever –Cararrhus Aestivus (Summer Cold)

John Bostock, M.D (1772–1846) presented an article in March of 1819 which is said to have been the first description of hay fever. In the article, he describes a patient (J.B) which turns out to be the author himself. In this case study he described the typical symptoms of allergic conjunctivitis, rhinitis and upper and lower airway symptoms including difficulty breathing. He noted the seasonality of the symptoms, which occurred yearly in June and abated by the end of July. The initial onset he approximated to have been at age 8. It is not clear by his writings if he was able to make the clear connection to pollens, but he does make the observation that remaining "nearly confined to the house for about 6 weeks...he experienced much less of the affection than he had done for several years before." Perhaps one of the first accounts of targeted exposure reduction to environmental allergens.[4]

Asthma–Allergy Connection

An early description of the unified airway concept and the association of asthma and allergy is provided by Blackley in his book *Experimental researches on the causes and nature of Catarrhus Aestivus (Hay-Fever or Hay-Asthma)* when describing his experiments involving challenging research subjects with pollen applied to the mucous membranes of the nose. He states "...there was also some oppression of breathing, which in this case must have been caused by reflex action, as there was, so far as I could judge, no pollen inhaled...I am satisfied that asthmatic symptoms may be brought on as hay-asthma by reflex action"[5]

Early Environmental Allergy Testing

Blackley is also known to have first described the process of skin testing for allergic reactions. Placing grains of pollen from grasses, trees, and weeds on the abraded skin of himself and his experimental subjects and observing the erythemic and urticarial reactions that followed. This along with the provocation testing described in his text (application of pollen to the mucous membranes) clearly linked the provoked respiratory symptoms with the suspected pollens.[5]

Early Descriptions of Food Allergy

Early mentions of probable food allergy also date back to Hippocrates as he described "hostile humors" or what we now know as immunoglobin E antibodies (IgE) that caused some individuals to "suffer badly" after ingesting cheese. The Roman poet and philosopher Titus Lucretius Carus (98–55 BCE), in his only known work, the philosophic poem *De rerum natura*, suggests that food allergy or adverse reactions to food were observed over 2000 years ago. His often quoted (sometimes incorrectly) line from that poem "*What is food to one, to another is rank poison*" describes the nature of type I hypersensitivity reactions.

The immunologic basis for food allergy however was first elucidated by an experiment reported by Carl Prausnitz (1876–1963) and Heinz Küstner (1897–1963) in

1921. Prausnitz injected serum from Küstner, who was allergic to fish, and a non-allergic control subject, into his own skin and a day later injected fish extract into the same areas. The positive local reaction in the area injected with Küstner's serum and not in the area from the negative control subject proved that sensitivity could be transferred by a substance (now identified as IgE) in the allergic patient's serum. This became known as a "Prausnitz- Küstner (P-K) reaction.[6]

Early Food Allergy Testing

In the early twentieth century, skin tests began to play a major role in identifying food allergens. Oscar M. Schloss, M.D (1892–1952) a physician and researcher in the United States performed some of the seminal work on food allergy diagnosis. In 1912 Dr. Schloss established the clinical practicability of performing scratch tests for clinical hypersensitivity to foods in controlled detailed studies. By utilizing the tuberculin abrasion technique introduced by Clemens von Pirquet (1879–1929) for investigating a child's rhinitis, asthma, and eczema, Schloss correlated cutaneous, erythematous wheal responses with clinically manifested "idiosyncrasies" to egg, almond, and oats.[7]

Allergy in the Twentieth Century–the Discovery of Immunoglobin E (IgE)

From the early work of researchers such as Prausnitz, Küstner, Schloss, and Von Pirquet it had become apparent that there were as yet unidentified substances that were responsible for type I sensitivity reactions. Von Pirquet described this as "supersensitivity without immunity" the properties of which included; inhalant allergy, immediately positive skin tests and the observation that other available tests for immunity were negative in these patients. In 1919 Maximillian Ramirez, M.D. reported in JAMA a case involving a previously non-allergic individual acquiring an allergy to horses after a blood transfusion from a horse-allergic individual. This was the first documented case of clinical allergy, not just sensitization, being transferred between individuals.[8]

It wasn't until the 1960's that investigators began in earnest to identify the substance that was responsible for P-K activity and type I hypersensitivity reactions. In Denver Colorado, Kimishige Ishizaka (1925–2018) and his wife Teruko Ishizaka (1926–2019) and their team analyzed sera from seasonal allergic rhinitis patients which had very high titers of P-K activity. Initial experiments suggested that the P-K activity was due to IgA, but this was later disproved by using a technology recently developed by Pharmacia a Swedish pharmaceutical and biotechnological company, of a cross-linked Sephadex separation medium G200 as a molecular sieve. Using this technique, they were able to separate the P-K activity from IgA. In 1966 they were able to produce an antiserum that could deplete P-K activity in serum and give a precipitin line in a gel. They went on to prove that this activity was not from IgA, IgM, IgG or the recently identified IgD. They suggested that this new isotype should be named gamma E.[8]

As is sometimes the case in science and medicine, discoveries are made contemporaneously by researchers in disparate locations of the planet. In Upsala Sweden Hans Bennich (1930-) and S. G. O. Johansson (1938-) developed an interest in a patient (ND) with multiple myeloma whose sera could not be typed as IgM, IgG, IgA or IgD. This patient's sera was ideal for study since it contained large quantities of myeloma protein. In 1967 working with two researchers in the UK, Bennich and Johansson digested the molecule with papain and determined that the Fc fragment could inhibit P-K activity. That year Ishizaka's group in Denver and the Upsala group exchanged reagents and it became clear that Ishizaka's purified P-K activity and the ND protein purified by Johansson and Bennich carried the same isotype-specific determinants. In 1968, the two groups presented their results and the official declaration of the new immunoglobulin class IgE was made by the World Health Organization Immunoglobulin Reference Center in Lausanne.[8,9]

In 1967 Johansson and Bennich along with a third scientist Leif Wide (1934-) also published a article describing the development of the radioallergosorbent test (RAST) for IgE antibodies. That article described how the assay was used to detect antibodies to 14 different allergens. Amazingly the researchers also reported a 96% agreement between results from provocation tests and this new test for allergic sensitization[10]

Pharmacia, whose role in identifying the IgE isotype with Sephadex was described earlier, would once again become a prominent force in allergy diagnostics as Johansson and colleagues went on to convince Pharmacia, later Phadia (Pharmacia Diagnostics) to collaborate in the development of assays for specific IgE antibodies and also those for the total quantity of IgE. A diagnostic group was formed and in 1972 the first commercial test for total IgE (Phadebas IgE) was introduced. In 1974 Phadebas RAST, using the "sandwich" technology developed by Leif Wide, was launched making the first time that it was possible for laboratories to measure IgE antibodies to specific allergens in serum. Continued improvements over the years saw RAST technology being supplanted with florescent enzyme-based technology and the paper disk solid phase being replaced with a three-dimensional cellulose sponge that allowed for markedly increased binding capacity. These improvements along with automation resulted in a reliable in vitro platform that facilitated widespread availability of accurate diagnostic testing for allergy-mediated diseases for both specialists and primary care clinicians alike.

1999 saw the commercial introduction of allergen components (mostly individual proteins) that allow for a more in-depth analysis than specific IgE whole allergen tests. Referred to as "molecular allergology" or "component resolved diagnosis" this constantly evolving area of allergy diagnosis, provides clinicians with an understanding of the characteristics of the individual allergen components to better predict the implications of specific sensitizations, allowing for a potentially more accurate diagnosis and personalized management approach. This topic can be explored further in Chapter 6 "Update on Allergy Diagnostics." Phadia now a subsidiary of Thermo Fisher Scientific continues to be the world leader in laboratory allergy diagnostics with widespread use and adoption of their ImmunoCAP brand of whole allergen and allergen component in vitro specific IgE assays.[11]

Asthma in the Twentieth Century

The beginning of the twentieth century found Sir William Osler (1849–1919) arguably one of the most influential physicians in history, discussing bronchial asthma in a chapter from his text published in 1901, *The Principals and Practices of Medicine*. While Osler's concept of asthma was similar to Henry Salter's discussed earlier, Osler went on to conclude that asthma was a psychoneurosis observing that both direct and psychogenic stimulation of the nervous system could provoke exacerbations. As a result, pharmacologic relief of anxiety was a mainstay of therapeutic interventions until the role of psychic stress was put into proper perspective in 1968.[12]

In 1917 Isaac Chandler Walker (1883–1950) of Peter Bent Brigham Hospital (later to become Brigham and Women's Hospital) in Boston, continued and advanced the correlation between asthma and allergy noting positive reactions with skin tests to proteins from animals, foods, and bacteria, in patients with asthma. While not all patients were sensitized to all tested substances, he was able to demonstrate a causal effect based on protein groupings and classified those patients accordingly.[13–15]

The phenotyping of asthma was first discussed by Francis Rackemann (1877–1973) who was the second president of the *Society for the study of Asthma and Allied Conditions* and the founder of the Allergy Clinic at Massachusetts General Hospital. Rackemann in his publication *A Clinical Study of One hundred fifty Cases of Bronchial Asthma*, published in 1918, confirmed the allergy asthma associations described by his fellow Bostonian Isaac Walker and referred to this as "extrinsic" causes of asthma. He further went on to describe non-allergic asthma as "intrinsic" and correlated this phenotype with other pathologic conditions found within the body. His investigations included very precise descriptions of skin testing techniques and correlation of the results with the individual clinical histories of each study subject. He grouped the extrinsic asthma patients by sensitizations including pollen asthma, horse asthma, and acute food asthma.[16]

Asthma Therapeutics

Pharmacologic and non-pharmacologic therapies for allergy and asthma have been employed for hundreds if not thousands of years. A mainstay of treatment for both allergy and allergic asthma has been the identification and avoidance of allergens to which a patient is sensitized. John Bostock, as described earlier in this chapter correlated his remaining indoors with a dramatic improvement in his seasonal allergic symptoms.[4] While allergen reduction and avoidance has proven to be a successful therapeutic intervention that has stood the test of time, there have been many other questionable or even dangerous interventions employed over the years. Therapeutic smoking was utilized as a therapy for asthma for hundreds of years. A variety of substances were employed including stramonium (an anticholinergic) which proved both dangerous and somewhat effective as well as cannabis sativa for its sedative and broncho-dilatory effects. Henry Salter was a proponent of smoking stramonium and recommended it not only for acute asthmatic exacerbations but also as a preventative measure specifically recommending to his patients, smoking a pipe each night before bed.[17]

The early twentieth century saw advice to change diet, move to or away from cities, live in the desert or at higher altitudes, sleep outdoors, and even hypnosis. Most of these had little if any effect.

In the 1920's better pharmacologic remedies began to emerge. In line with Henry Salter's recommendation for hot strong coffee (described earlier) research began into other xanthines. In 1921 researchers Macht and Ting confirmed that xanthines relaxed smooth muscle and theophylline suppositories were first used in 1922 to treat asthma. Aminophylline entered our armamentarium in 1937 and along with theophylline remained key treatments until the 1980's.

Although experiencing a slower rate of adoption, sympathomimetics use preceded the xanthines but didn't really gain prominence until they were demonstrated to be more efficacious, with a wider therapeutic window than the xanthines. Epinephrine, first administered in 1903 and later isoproterenol (1949) administered by both injection and inhalation were demonstrated to have rapid, quite effective broncho-dilatory effects. Both medications although effective had troublesome cardiac and systemic side effects.[18] Inhalation devices such as atomizers developed in 1849 and nebulizers shortly thereafter in 1862 were utilized to deliver many of the early therapeutics.[19]

1956 saw the invention of the multi-dose inhaler and the subsequent introduction of numerous adrenergic medications with continuous improvements involving β-2 adrenergic selectivity resulting in less troublesome side effects, and increased durations of action. Concurrently anti-cholinergics experienced a resurgence, remember stramonium, but now without the need to "smoke it." The atropine molecule was modified, and ipratropium was introduced in 1975. Long-acting beta agonists such as salmeterol and formoterol arrived on the scene but concerns about their contribution to "loss of control" and deaths when administered as monotherapy has limited their use to therapeutic combinations with inhaled corticosteroids. Long-acting muscarinic (anticholinergics) have recently gained favor in the treatment of certain asthma phenotypes. Treatment up until 1956 was only focused on addressing the spasmodic component of asthma, but in 1956 systemic glucocorticoids were first introduced for both acute and chronic asthma directed specifically at airway inflammation. Systemic side effects limited their chronic use until the introduction of inhaled preparations (beclomethasone and betamethasone.) Improvements in the potency and duration of action soon led to the adoption of inhaled corticosteroids as first-line treatments for persistent asthma.[12]

Systemic steroids remained the only available option for severe/uncontrolled asthma until the introduction of omalizumab, an anti-IgE therapeutic in 2003. This was followed by 5 additional biologics introduced from 2015 to 2021. These medications generally target cytokines directly involved in the pathology of severe asthma, leading to a reduction in oral corticosteroid use and measurable decreases in severe exacerbations.[18]

Allergy Therapeutics

Histamine was identified in 1907 and by 1910 had been isolated from bacterial fermentation. In 1937 the first antihistamine was developed by the Nobel prize winning chemist Daniel Bovet (1907–1992.) The first commercially available antihistamine was Antergan (dimethylethylene diamine.) Other first-generation H-1 antagonists followed. Diphenhydramine was discovered in 1943 by George Rieveschl, a professor at the University of Cincinnati. In 1946, it became the first prescription antihistamine approved by the FDA.[20] The first generation (mepyramine, dimetindene, clemastine, diphenhydramine, and so forth) had considerable sedative side effects. The second-generation antihistamines starting with terfenadine and loratadine demonstrated much less sedation and the third-generation antihistamines such as fexofenadine, levocetirizine, and desloratadine even less.[1]

Decongestants, both topical and systemic, were used adjunctively to address congestion related to nasal mucosal swelling. Intranasal antihistamines, mast cell stabilizers, and leukotriene receptor antagonists all expanded the available treatment options throughout the latter half of the twentieth century. Inhaled nasal corticosteroids (INS) were introduced in the 1950's and progressed throughout the 1970's and 80's. In 1987 the Montreal Protocol, which phased out chlorofluorocarbon propellants due to their environmental effects on the ozone layer, significantly limited INS treatment options to only aqueous options until the approval of the first hydrofluoroalkane propellant for intra-nasal steroids in 2012. Combination INS products (corticosteroid/antihistamine) were introduced more recently and have demonstrated increased efficacy over single-agent therapeutics.[19,20]

Allergen Immunotherapy

Leonard Noon (1877–1913) and his colleague John Freeman (1877–1962) working in St. Mary's Hospital, London, first described the use of allergen immunotherapy in separate publications in 1911. *Prophylactic inoculation against hay fever* and *Further observations of the treatment of hay fever by hypodermic inoculations of pollen vaccine.* Noon and colleagues used conjunctival provocation testing to demonstrate protection after grass pollen extract exposure. Noon unfortunately died of tuberculosis shortly thereafter, leaving Freeman to carry on their collaborative work.[21,22]

After the publication of these seminal research articles, the use of allergen immuno-therapy (AIT) accelerated worldwide for the treatment of "hay fever" patients. But it wasn't until the 1950's when the first double-blind, placebo-controlled trial was per-formed. William Frankland (1912–2020) in England, who had worked with John Freeman published results of the first controlled trial proving that hypersensitization was significantly more effective in higher doses than in a lower dose or when using pla-cebo in the treatment of hay fever. In 1978 the first randomized, double-blinded, pla-cebo-controlled, trial (RDBPC) for AIT in the treatment of hymenoptera venom allergy was performed and confirmed the utility of using purified venoms over whole body extracts.

While subcutaneous immunotherapy (SCIT) has been the standard since for over one hundred years, other routes such as sublingual immunotherapy (SLIT) have gained acceptance for the treatment of environmental allergies more recently. The first RDBPC trial for SLIT was published in 1986 and was quickly followed by other studies that confirmed its efficacy.[22]

While SLIT was utilized "off-label" since the 1980's, in 2014 the FDA approved the first sublingual tablet product for use in the United States. Initially for grass pollen al-lergy, other products for ragweed and dust mite eventually also gained approval.[23]

Oral immunotherapy specifically for food allergy had its origins in the early 1900's but the first published study demonstrating efficacy was in 1984 when Patriarca pub-lished *Oral specific hyposensitization in the management of patients allergic to food*. In January 2020 the FDA approved the first oral immunotherapy for peanut allergy Pal-forzia. Other methods of desensitization for food allergy have been and are currently being explored, such as transdermal immunotherapy.[24]

SUMMARY

The history of both allergy and asthma has been intertwined since their earliest de-scriptions. It is therefore easy to see why these two conditions are often discussed and studied together. Improvements in the diagnosis and management of these mal-adies continues to be made and like many areas of science and medicine will no doubt increase exponentially in the twenty-first century.

DISCLOSURE

G. Falcetano is an employee of Thermo Fisher Scientific, a biotechnology company that manufactures diagnostic laboratory instruments both allergy and autoimmune disorders.

REFERENCES

1. Ring J. History of Allergy: Clinical Descriptions, Pathophysiology, and Treatment. In: Traidl-Hoffmann C, Zuberbier T, Werfel T, editors. Allergic diseases – from basic mechanisms to comprehensive management and prevention . Handbook of experimental pharmacology268. Cham: Springer; 2021. https://doi.org/10.1007/164_2021_509.

2. Marketos SG, Ballas CN. Bronchial asthma in the medical literature of Greek an-tiquity. J Asthma 1982;19(4):263–9.

3. Sakula A. Henry Hyde Salter (1823-71): a biographical sketch. Thorax 1985 Dec; 40(12):887–8 [Erratum in: Thorax 1986 May;41(5):416].

4. Ramachandran M. John Bostock's first description of hay fever. J R Soc Med 2011;104:237–40.

5. Blackley C. Experiments and researches on the causes of nature of catarrhus aestivus. London: Balliere, Tindall & Cox; 1873.
6. Sampson HA. Food allergy: Past, present and future. Allergol Int 2016;65(Issue 4):363–9.
7. Cohen SG. Food allergens: landmarks along a historic trail. J Allergy Clin Immunol 2008;121(6):1521–4.
8. Platts-Mills TA, Heymann PW, Commins SP, et al. The discovery of IgE 50 years later. Ann Allergy Asthma Immunol 2016;116(3):179–82.
9. Johansson SG. The discovery of immunoglobulin e and its role in allergy. Chem Immunol Allergy 2014;100:150–4.
10. Wide L, Bennich H, Johansson SG. Diagnosis of allergy by an in-vitro test for allergen antibodies. Lancet 1967;2(7526):1105–7.
11. Our history Available at: http://www.phadia.com/en/About-us/Phadia-History/.
12. McFadden ER Jr. A century of asthma. Am J Respir Crit Care Med 2004;170(3):215–21.
13. Walker C. Studies on the sensitization of patients with bronchial asthma to bacterial proteins as demonstrated by the skin reaction and the methods employed in the preparation of these proteins. J Med Res 1917;35:487–95.
14. Walker C. Studies on the sensitization of patients with bronchial asthma to the different proteins found in the dandruff of the horse and in the hair of the cat and the dog and to the sera of these animals. J Med Res 1917;35:497–508.
15. Walker C. Studies on the sensitization of patients with bronchial asthma to the different proteins in wheat and to the whole protein of wheat, corn, rice, barley, rye, and oat. J Med Res 1917;35:509–13.
16. Rackemann FM. A clinical study of one hundred fifty cases of bronchial asthma. Arch Intern Med 1918;22:552.
17. Jackson M. "Divine stramonium": the rise and fall of smoking for asthma. Med Hist 2010;54(2):171–94.
18. Sutherby RA. Surge of Biologics for Severe Asthma. Managed Healthcare Executive MHE June 2022;32:6.
19. Stein SW, Thiel CG. The History of Therapeutic Aerosols: A Chronological Review. J Aerosol Med Pulm Drug Deliv 2017;30(1):20–41.
20. Ostrom NK. The history and progression of treatments for allergic rhinitis. Allergy Asthma Proc 2014;35(Suppl 1):S3–10.
21. Ring J, Gutermuth J. 100 years of hypo sensitization: history of allergen-specific immunotherapy (ASIT). Allergy 2011;66:713–24.
22. Passalacqua G, Canonica GW. Allergen Immunotherapy: History and Future Developments. Immunol Allergy Clin North Am 2016;36(1):1–12.
23. Passalacqua G, Bagnasco D, Canonica GW. 30 years of sublingual immunotherapy. Allergy 2020;75(5):1107–20.
24. Dunlop JH. Oral immunotherapy for treatment of peanut allergy. J Investig Med 2020;68(6):1152–5.

Basic Immunology and Primary Immunodeficiency

Amanda Michaud, DMSc, PA-C, AE-C[a],*, Jennifer Watson, MN, FNP-C[b]

KEYWORDS

- Immunology • Primary immune deficiency • Immunodeficiency • Immune system
- Gamma globulin

KEY POINTS

- Primary immunodeficiencies (PIDDs) are inherited disorders that result in immune dysregulation and can predispose patients to recurrent and severe infections.
- Immunodeficiency should be suspected in any patient with recurrent bacterial infections or other warning signs of PIDD.
- The diagnostic evaluation for PIDD varies. Initial evaluation typically includes complete blood count and differential, quantitative immunoglobulins, and evaluating for specific antibody responses.
- Other conditions that could contribute to recurrent infections or immunodeficiency must be ruled out before diagnosis of PIDD is made.
- Management depends on the PIDD identified and the severity and frequency of infections. Treatment may include stem cell transplant, prophylactic antibiotics or antifungals, and replacement immunoglobulin infusions, among others.

THE IMMUNE SYSTEM
Introduction

The immune system involves an assortment of chemicals and cells that work to protect the body from foreign antigens, including viruses, microbes, toxins, and cancer.[1,2] There are two general parts of the immune system, referred to as the innate and adaptive immune systems. The innate immune system is the body's first line of defense against a pathogen. The innate immune system is a general (nonspecific) immune system that is activated immediately after encountering a foreign antigen. There is no "memory" associated with the innate immune system, so it is unable to recognize the same foreign antigen on subsequent exposure.[1] Unlike the general innate immune system, the adaptive immune system is antigen-specific.[1,3,4] The adaptive immune

[a] Family Allergy and Asthma Consultants, 4123 University Boulevard South, Suite B, Jacksonville, FL 32216, USA; [b] Asthma & Allergy of Idaho, 714 West Appleway Suite 200, Coeur d'Alene, ID 83814, USA
* Corresponding author.
E-mail address: amandalmichaud@gmail.com

Physician Assist Clin 8 (2023) 621–632
https://doi.org/10.1016/j.cpha.2023.05.001
2405-7991/23/© 2023 Elsevier Inc. All rights reserved.

system has immunologic memory, which allows a more efficient and specific response when the body is exposed to a particular antigen it has encountered previously. The adaptive immune system responds after a delay, but with a more appropriate, targeted response to the foreign antigen. The innate and active immune systems work together to protect the host.

The Innate Immune System

The innate immune system has various types of defensive barriers, including the skin, mucous membranes, temperature, low pH, chemical mediators, and various phagocytic and inflammatory barriers.[1] Barriers, such as the skin, help to obstruct the entry of microbes, whereas the low pH of the stomach can help kill microbes. Other barriers include elevated body temperature (fever), which can prevent pathogen growth, and specialized immune cells that can break down and phagocytose organisms or activate other defenses. A major part of the innate immune system is the rapid activation of various immune cells.[1–3] Cytokines and chemokines are responsible for communication between cells and recruitment of other immune cells. This communication can summon a variety of other immune cells to help clear a particular pathogen. Various cells involved in the innate immune system include phagocytes (macrophages and neutrophils), mast cells, basophils, eosinophils, natural killer cells, dendritic cells, and innate lymphoid cells. These various cells and their features and functions are noted in **Fig. 1**.

The Adaptive Immune System

The adaptive immune system's processes are partly assisted by the innate immune system.[1,4] The adaptive immune system has a critical role in eliminating infectious pathogens. Its main functions are to recognize and distinguish antigens, and produce specific immune pathways to eliminate various pathogens. Finally, the adaptive immune system also develops the immunologic "memory" that allows the immune system to swiftly eradicate a specific pathogen in the future on subsequent exposure or reinfection. The main cells of the adaptive immune system include antigen-specific T cells, antigen-presenting cells (APCs), and B cells. B cells are able to further separate into plasma cells to create antibodies.

T cells are produced by stem cells in the bone marrow and mature in the thymus gland.[4] Each T cell has unique receptors and is able to rapidly activate and be involved in different processes when signaled to do so. When given the proper signal from an APC, the T cell is activated and helps to regulate the immune response. T cells then

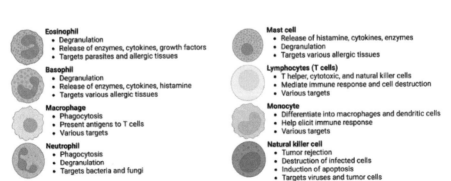

Fig. 1. Types and function of cells involved in innate immunity.[1–3] (Created with BioRender. com.)

differentiate into either cytotoxic T cells (function to destroy cells infected by various pathogens), or T-helper cells (function to active macrophages and B-cell multiplication via cytokine release). B cells can then multiply and mature into plasma cells that produce antibodies. These antibodies target and bind to various pathogens, which then "flags" them for destruction by other immune cells.[1,4] Once the pathogen is eliminated, the antigen-antibody complex is destroyed by the complement system. Without the adaptive immune system, the innate immune system is unable to clear infections.[5] A simplified comparison of the innate versus adaptive immune systems is seen in **Fig. 2**.

The Complement System

The complement system refers to a sequence of events that functions to identify and alter bacteria and other pathogens to make them easier to eradicate.[5] This allows the innate immune system to phagocytize microbes and kill pathogens, while also helping the adaptive immune system mobilize and activate APCs more easily. Antigen-antibody complexes are eliminated by the complement system.

IMMUNODEFICIENCY

When the immune system's ability to fight infections is compromised or absent, this is referred to as immunodeficiency. Primary immunodeficiency disorders (PIDDs) result from genetic or inherited defects, whereas secondary immunodeficiency disorders result because of another, secondary cause, such as an autoimmune condition, immunosuppressive medication use, or various cancers.[6] People with immunodeficiency disorders are at increased risk of recurrent and possibly serious viral, bacterial, and fungal infections. More than 350 PIDDs have been identified.[7] PIDDs are typically classified according to the clinical features, such as types of infections seen, and which part of the immune system is disrupted. Disorders of adaptive immunity include B-cell (antibody-mediated), T-cell (cellular-mediated), and combined (B- and T-cell) immunodeficiencies.[5,7,8] Disorders of innate immunity include phagocyte and complement defects. Many of the different types of PIDDs are outlined in **Table 1**.

T-cell immunodeficiencies are recognized as among the most severe immunodeficiencies.[5,7] Because T cells are required for B-cell maturation, T-cell deficiencies also

Innate immunity (quick, non-specific)

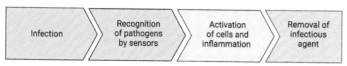

Adaptive immunity (long-term, specific)

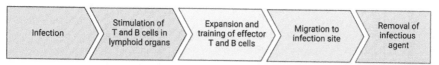

Fig. 2. Innate and adaptive immunity. The immune system protects the host from invading pathogens through two layers: the innate and adaptive immune systems. Innate immunity acts within minutes to remove the pathogen. Adaptive immunity takes longer (days or weeks) but is antigen-specific and long-lasting. (Created with BioRender.com.)

Table 1
PIDD types and various clinical presentations[5,7,8]

	Types of PIDD and Examples	Various Presentations
Combined immunodeficiencies	• Severe combined immunodeficiency • Other combined immunodeficiencies with low CD4, low CD8, normal/low immunoglobulins, or poor specific antibody responses • Combined immunodeficiencies associated with syndromes	• Recurrent and/or severe bacterial and viral infections • Opportunistic infections common • Diarrhea • Failure to thrive • Dermatitis or eczema • Cardiac abnormalities • Thrombocytopenia • Ataxia • Autoimmune disease
Predominantly antibody defects	• X-linked agammaglobulinemia • Common variable immunodeficiency • IgA deficiency • Genetic hypogammaglobulinemias • Hyper-IgM syndromes • Transient hypogammaglobulinemia of infancy • IgG subclass deficiency • Specific antibody deficiency	• Recurrent bacterial sinopulmonary infections • Autoimmune disease may be present • Increased risk of malignancy in some conditions, such as common variable immunodeficiency
Phagocyte defects	• Chronic granulomatous disease • G6PD deficiency • GATA2 deficiency • Shwachman–Diamond syndrome	• Severe infections • Abscess and granuloma formation • Poor wound healing
Complement defects	• Deficiency in early or late complement components • Deficiency of other complement regulatory proteins	• Autoimmune diseases • Recurrent infections
Other defects in intrinsic or innate immunity	• Chronic mucocutaneous candidiasis • Congenital asplenia • IRAK1 or IRAK4 deficiency • Interferon-gamma receptor defects	• Splenomegaly • Adenopathy • Rashes • Autoimmune conditions • Cytopenias • Dental hypoplasia

lead to some B-cell deficiency. T-cell deficiency usually presents early in life, within the first 6 to 12 months of life, after waning of protective maternal antibodies. Newborn screening for T-cell receptor excision circles has been adopted in all states and has allowed early detection of T-cell deficiencies, which is fatal if led untreated.[5,9] Hematopoietic stem cell transplant is necessary for treatment. Severe combined immunodeficiency (SCID) occurs when there are defects in all types of lymphocytes. This is also typically diagnosed at birth via screening or in early infancy because of recurrent and severe infections in early life.

Antibody deficiencies, also known as B-cell deficiencies, are the most common types of PIDD, accounting for approximately half of all cases.[5,8] Depending on the type of antibody deficiency, these can present early in life or in adulthood.[5] These immunodeficiencies typically present with recurrent bacterial infections, typically affecting the sinopulmonary tract, and involving pyogenic bacteria. Examples of antibody deficiencies include X-linked agammaglobulinemia (XLA), common variable immune deficiency (CVID), selective IgA deficiency, and specific antibody deficiency.[5,10] XLA, also known as Bruton agammaglobulinemia, has an absence of B cells, which results in very low immunoglobulin levels.[5] IgA deficiency is the most common antibody deficiency, in which patients have low IgA. Some patients with IgA deficiency fortunately do not suffer from recurrent infections. CVID presents with low immunoglobulin levels and recurrent infections. Finally, patients with specific antibody deficiency have normal antibody and immunoglobulin levels, but lack proper antibody response to specific vaccine antigens.[10]

Complement deficiencies are rare and occur when patients have defects in components of the complement cascade that are important in the function of the immune system.[5] Patients with phagocyte deficiencies are at increased risk of bacterial and opportunistic infections. There have been numerous other immunodeficiencies identified but full discussion is beyond the scope of this review.

Secondary immunodeficiency can also cause recurrent infections and present with similar symptoms as primary immunodeficiency, but are far more common.[6,11] Secondary immunodeficiency can result because of other abnormal immune function related to malignancy, infectious diseases (eg, certain viral infections or HIV/AIDS), malnutrition, or because of various immunosuppressive medications.[11,12] Other issues, such as chronic stress and sleep deprivation, can contribute to development of secondary immunodeficiency. Therefore, when evaluating for immunodeficiency, the clinician must be aware of and rule out secondary causes. A list of different causes of secondary immunodeficiency is found in **Box 1**.

CLINICAL PRESENTATION

PIDD can occur at any age. PIDD should be considered in patients with recurrent, unusual, or persistent infections.[8] PIDD should be considered if any of the following are present, as noted in **Fig. 3**: (1) unusual site of infections, (2) unusual frequency of infections, (3) unusual pathogens or opportunistic infections, (4) syndromic features are present, (5) presence of autoimmune disease or malignancy, (6) a family history of PIDD, and (7) unusual severity of infections.[12] **Box 2** lists warning signs of PIDD, and patients with any of these criteria should be referred for evaluation for PIDD with a clinical immunologist.[13]

Most often, patients with PIDD present with recurrent otitis and/or sinopulmonary infections.[7,8] PIDD should also be suspected if routine illnesses become more complicated and lead to sepsis, meningitis, or other infections.[8] PIDDs can also present as recurrent cutaneous and gastrointestinal infections. For certain PIDDs that involve

> **Box 1**
> **Causes of secondary immunodeficiency[6,11,12]**
>
> - HIV/AIDS
> - Malignancy
> - Malnutrition
> - Immunosuppressive medications
>   - Corticosteroids
>   - Calcineurin inhibitors
>   - Cytotoxic agents
>   - Biologics
>   - Antiepileptics
> - Genetic disorder
>   - Trisomy 21
>   - Turner syndrome
>   - Cystic fibrosis
> - Metabolic disorders
>   - Diabetes mellitus
>   - Nephrotic syndrome
>   - Protein-losing enteropathy
>
> Autoimmune conditions
>
> - Autoinflammatory conditions

T-cell or combined B- and T-cell dysfunction, patients can present with failure to thrive, facial dysmorphia, ectodermal dysplasia, congenital heart disease, recurrent viral infections, autoimmune diseases, or chronic diarrhea.[7,8] Patients with SCID typically present before 1 year of age with chronic diarrhea, failure to thrive, and severe infections. SCID is fatal if not identified and treated, but thankfully the United States has instituted newborn screening for SCID in all 50 states since 2018.[9] Antibody deficiencies typically present with recurrent bacterial sinopulmonary infections, poor response to immunizations, and autoimmune disease.[8] Recurrent pulmonary infections occur in 80% of patients with antibody deficiencies.[14] Patients with T-cell defects may present with recurrent and potentially severe viral infections, recurrent fungal infection or oral thrush, recurrent bacterial infections, mycobacterial infections, chronic diarrhea, and failure to thrive.[15] Complement defects may present with recurrent infections and autoimmune disease, whereas phagocyte defects may present

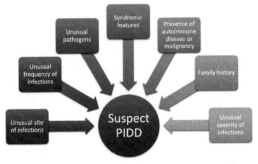

Fig. 3. Features of PIDD that should raise suspicion for diagnosis.[12]

Box 2
Warning signs of PIDD, from the Jeffrey Modell Foundation[13]

Warning signs in children:
1. ≥4 new ear infections within 1 year
2. ≥2 serious sinus infections within 1 year
3. ≥2 months of antibiotic course with little improvement
4. ≥2 pneumonias within 1 year
5. Failure of an infant to grow normally or gain weight
6. Recurrent, deep skin or organ abscesses
7. Persistent thrush in mouth or fungal infection of the skin
8. Need for intravenous antibiotics to clear infections
9. ≥2 deep-seated infections including septicemia
10. A family history of PIDD

Warning signs in adults:
1. ≥2 new ear infections within 1 year
2. ≥2 new sinus infections within 1 year, in the absence of allergy
3. 1 pneumonia per year for greater than 1 year
4. Chronic diarrhea with weight loss
5. Recurrent viral infections (eg, upper respiratory infections, warts)
6. Recurrent, deep abscesses of the skin or internal organs
7. Recurrent need for intravenous antibiotics to clear infections
8. Persistent thrush in mouth or fungal infection of the skin
9. Infection with normally harmless tuberculosis-like bacteria
10. A family history of PIDD

with recurrent viral infections and atypical mycobacterial infections. Patients with PIDD affecting their neutrophils may present with recurrent abscesses, granulomas, or pneumonias. Patients with chronic deep-seated infections, such as deep abscesses or recurrent osteomyelitis, should raise concern for chronic granulomatous disease (CGD).[7] Presentations of PIDDs are highly variable, with many patients also presenting with more severe infections, such as sepsis, meningitis, hepatitis, or various malignancies. A detailed history should be taken, including key elements, such as duration of illnesses, onset of recurrent infections, presence of constitutional symptoms, history of underlying lung disease or autoimmune conditions, and family history.[14]

The physical examination in patients with PIDD may be normal, because patients may or may not seem ill. On physical examination, patients may have lymphadenopathy; splenomegaly; skin rashes; and in some cases, absence of tonsils.[6,8,16] Skin rashes can include maculopapular eruptions, pyoderma, eczema, petechiae, telangiectasias, warts, vitiligo, or alopecia.[16,17] Examination of the head and neck may reveal evidence of allergic rhinitis or chronic sinusitis.[16] The ears should be examined for otitis media, and oropharynx evaluated for signs of infection or presence of ulcers. Examination of the ears may also reveal scarred or perforated tympanic membranes, secondary to recurrent infections.[8] Cervical lymphoid tissue and tonsillar/adenoid tissue are often absent in certain conditions, such as XLA, hyper-IgM syndrome, or SCID.[8,17] However, in other conditions, such as CGD, cervical lymph nodes may be enlarged.[16] Patients with PIDD may present with signs of pulmonary infection, such as rhonchi or rales.[14] Hepatosplenomegaly can also be seen in CVID or CGD.[7,8] When evaluating a patient for PIDD, it is also important to note the patient's weight and height and assess for failure to thrive.[7] Delayed diagnosis is common, unfortunately leading to increased infections, recurrent hospitalizations, and increased health care costs.

DIAGNOSIS
Laboratory Studies

Blood tests are necessary to evaluate for underlying PIDD. Initial work-up includes a complete blood count with differential, quantitative immunoglobulins (IgA, IgG, IgM, and IgE), and specific antibody titers to immunizations.[8,14,16] Complete blood count with a differential is performed to assess for lymphopenia, unusual lymphocytes or other phagocytic cells, or other abnormalities associated with PIDDs. Newborn T-cell receptor excision circles screens allows for evaluation of T cells and can identify most cases of SCID in newborns.[8,9]

Assessment of antibody titers includes those for diphtheria, tetanus, *Streptococcus pneumoniae*, and *Haemophilus influenzae* B, and sometimes naturally occurring antibodies because of other infections.[7,15] For T-cell defects, lymphocyte subsets along with functional assays, including mitogens or antigens, are important.[7,8,15]

For antibody deficiencies, assessing pneumococcal titers and response to vaccination with a pneumococcal polysaccharide vaccine (eg, PPSV23) reveals absent or partial response.[7,10] B cells and T cells are evaluated via flow cytometry and may be absent or severely reduced in SCID, CVID, agammaglobulinemia, and other PIDD conditions.[7,8,10] T-helper-cell function can also be assessed by assessing the protein-based antigens, such as tetanus. Deficiencies of the complement system can initially be evaluated with total complement (referred to as CH50). Further work-up and other laboratory tests may be necessary depending on the clinical presentation and suspected PIDD. **Table 2** is a summary of the various laboratory tests used in diagnosis for PIDD, along with their various abnormalities and some of the possible related immune defects.

Radiographic Studies

Radiographic studies are useful in detecting clinical manifestations of PIDD, but have minimal role in specific diagnosis. In infants, an absence of the thymus may indicate SCID.[16] Abdominal imaging is done to evaluate for abscesses, hepatosplenomegaly, lymphoid hyperplasia, and granulomatous disease of the gastrointestinal tract.[7,15] Chest imaging is done to assess for active pneumonia or infection, granulomatous disease of the lungs, bronchiectasis, or presence of other lung disease.[7,14]

MANAGEMENT

Management of PIDDs is complex and should be performed under the care of an immunology team. For B-cell immunodeficiencies, replacement immunoglobulin is standard of care and administered either intravenously or subcutaneously.[7,8] Most patients require replacement immunoglobulin infusions for life. The recommended starting dose of replacement therapy is 400 to 600 mg/kg/month. There are numerous products with various concentrations and infusion rates available, with flexibility for patients to have weekly, biweekly, or monthly infusions. In some cases, patients may warrant more conservative treatment and not require replacement gamma globulin infusions, such as in some patients with selective IgA deficiency or specific antibody deficiency.[4,7,8]

Antimicrobial prophylaxis is recommended for patients with certain PIDDs and may be used in patients with antibody deficiencies as an adjuvant to immunoglobulin replacement.[8] Antifungal prophylaxis is also recommended for patients with CGD. Live vaccines should be avoided in PIDD, especially in patients with severe T-cell defects or severe agammaglobulinemia.[7] In children with SCID, stem cell transplants or bone marrow transplants is life-saving.[6] Bone marrow transplantation has also been performed in patients with other immune defects, such as CGD. Gene therapy is an

Table 2
Laboratory evaluation and abnormalities of various types of PIDDs[1,5,7–10]

Laboratory Test	Abnormality	Possible Immune Defect
Complete blood count with differential	Lymphopenia Thrombocytopenia Eosinophilia	SCID Congenital neutropenia Wiskott-Aldrich syndrome
Neutrophil oxidative burst assay	Absent	CGD
Total complement (CH50) and other complement components	Negative	Complement deficiency
T-cell markers	Low	Multiple immunodeficiencies, including SCID, CVID, and other antibody deficiencies
B-cell markers	Absent mature B cells with or without absent or low T cells or natural killer cells	XLA SCID
IgG	Low or absent	XLA Hyper-IgM syndrome CVID SCID
IgA	Low or absent	Selective IgA deficiency CVID
IgM	Elevated or low/absent	Hyper-IgM syndrome CVID
IgE	Elevated	Hyper-IgE syndrome
Specific antibody titers	Nonprotective or absent, with poor response on vaccination	Various antibody deficiencies
Lymphocyte stimulation by mitogens	Absent	SCID DiGeorge syndrome

emerging treatment option for some types of PIDD.[8] **Fig. 4** summarizes the diagnosis and management of PIDD.

The risk of infection is high for those with underlying PIDD. Therefore, it is important to avoid unnecessary infection exposures and for patients to be up to date on vaccinations. Aggressive management of any infection is imperative. In the event of infection, identification of the causative organism is helpful and recommended. An awareness of autoimmune disease and malignancy must also be kept in mind, because those with underlying immunodeficiency are at a higher risk of these conditions.[5,7,8] Finally, genetic counseling is essential for families of patients with PIDD.[17]

DISCUSSION

PIDDs should be suspected in patients with recurrent and/or unusual infections, or those with a family history of PIDD. There have been more than 350 different PIDDs identified with various presentations, but the most common presentation is recurrent infection. There is often delayed diagnosis of many PIDDs because of lack of clinician awareness of the warning signs of PIDD. PIDD can present at any age. Thankfully,

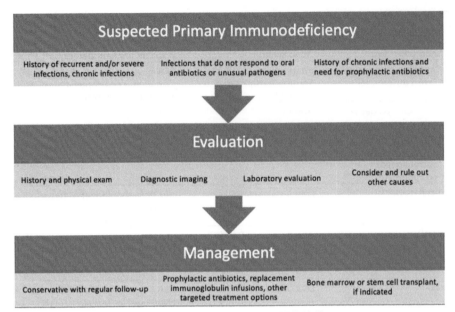

Fig. 4. Evaluation and management of suspected PIDD.[5,7,12,14,16]

improved newborn screening has allowed detection and prompt management of potentially life-threatening T-cell deficiencies. Patients with PIDD can also present with complex clinical syndromes, autoimmune disorders, atopic conditions, and malignancy, which adds to the complexity of their diagnosis and management. Because of the complex nature of these conditions, these patients should be referred to the immunology clinic for evaluation and management. Most patients with PIDDs require immunoglobulin replacement to protect them from recurrent infections, and some may require prophylactic antibiotic and antifungal treatment to further prevent infections.

SUMMARY

PIDDs are rare disorders that can cause recurrent and severe infections. Clinicians must be aware of the warning signs of PIDD and when to refer patients to clinical immunologists for proper evaluation of recurrent infections. Diagnosis of PIDDs is often delayed, and early detection and proper management can improve morbidity and mortality associated with PIDDs. Antibiotics or antifungal prophylaxis, immunoglobulin replacement, early recognition of infection, and at times, hematopoietic stem cell transplant or bone marrow transplant can save lives, help prevent infections and end-organ damage, and improve long-term outcomes and quality of life.

RESOURCES FOR CLINICIANS

- Immune Deficiency Foundation - www.primaryimmune.org
- American Academy of Allergy, Asthma, and Immunology - www.aaaai.org
- Clinical Immunology Society - www.clinimmsoc.org
- European Society for Immunodeficiencies - www.esid.org
- Jeffrey Modell Foundation/Primary Immunodeficiency Resource Center - www.info4pi.org
- US Immunodeficiency Network - www.usidnet.org

CLINICS CARE POINTS

- PIDD should be suspected in patients with recurrent, unusual, or difficult-to-treat infection history.
- Clinicians must be aware of the warning signs of PIDD and their various presentations.
- Initial work-up of patients with suspected PIDD involves complete blood count with differential, quantitative immunoglobulins, and evaluation of specific vaccine responses.
- Most patients with PIDD require immunoglobulin-replacement therapy.
- Early recognition, diagnosis, and management can improve outcomes in patients with PIDD.

DISCLOSURE

The authors have no commercial financial conflicts of interest pertinent to the topic. No funding sources have been allotted for the publication of this article.

REFERENCES

1. Marshall JS, Warrington R, Watson W, et al. An introduction to immunology and immunopathology. Allergy Asthma Clin Immunol 2018;14(2):49.
2. Murphy K, Weaver C, Berg LJ. Janeway's immunobiology. 10th edition. New York, NY: WW Norton and Company Publishing; 2022.
3. Turvey SE, Broide DH. Innate immunity. J Allergy Clin Immunol 2010;125(Supp 2): S24–32.
4. Bonilla FA, Oettgen HC. Adaptive immunity. J Allergy Clin Immunol 2010; 125(Supp 2):S33–40.
5. Immunodeficiency. In: Levinson W, Chin-Hong P, Joyce EA, et al, editors. Review of Medical Microbiology and Immunology: a guide to clinical infectious diseases. 17th edition. New York, NY: McGraw Hill; 2022. p. 589–94. Available at: https:// accessmedicine-mhmedical-com.ezproxy.lynchburg.edu/content.aspx?bookid= 3123&sectionid=262002080. Accessed October 22, 2022.
6. Bonilla FA, Bernstein IL, Khan DA, et al. Practice parameter for the diagnosis and management of primary immunodeficiency. Ann Allergy Asthma Immunol 2005; 94:S1–63.
7. Spickett G. Primary immunodeficiency. In: Spickett G, editor. Oxford handbook of clinical immunology and allergy. 4th edition. New York, NY: Oxford University Press; 2020. p. 3–88.
8. McCusker C, Upton J, Warrington R. Primary immunodeficiency. Allergy Asthma Clin Immunol 2018;14(2):61.
9. Currier R, Puck JM. SCID newborn screening: what we've learned. J Allergy Clin Immunol 2021;147(2):417–26.
10. Uzzaman A, Fuleihan RL. Approach to primary immunodeficiency. Allergy Asthma Proc 2012;33:S91–5.
11. Hausman O, Warnatz K. Immunodeficiency in adults: a practical guide for the allergist. Allergo J Int 2014;23:261–8.
12. Murali MR. Approach to recurrent infections in adults. In DynaMed database on-line. EBSCO Information Services. Available at: https://www.dynamed.com/ approach-to/approach-to-recurrent-infectionsin-adults#ANATOMIC _CAUSES_ OF_RECURRENT_INFECTIONS_IN_ADULTS. Updated August 10, 2016. Accessed October 23, 2022.

13. Jeffrey Modell Foundation. Primary immunodeficiency resource center. Available at: http://www.info4pi.org/library/educational-materials/10-warning-signs. Accessed October 1, 2022.
14. Cunningham-Rundles C. Evaluating the adult with recurrent infections. In: Sampson HA, editor. Mount sinai expert guides: allergy and clinical immunology. Hoboken, NJ: Wiley Blackwell Publishing; 2015. p. 335–40.
15. Forbes L, Brown-Whitehorn T. Approach to the child with immunodeficiency. In: Florin T, Aronson P, Werner H, et al, editors. Netter's pediatrics. 1st edition. Philadelphia, PA: Elsevier; 2011. p. 124–31.
16. Agarwal S. Evaluating the child with recurrent infections. In: Sampson HA, editor. Mount sinai expert guides: allergy and clinical immunology. Wiley Blackwell Publishing; 2015. p. 327–34.
17. Buckley RH, editor. Diagnostic and clinical care guidelines for primary immunodeficiency diseases. 3rd edition. Towson, MD: Immune Deficiency Foundation; 2015.

Not Just a Disease of the Nose

Allergic Rhinitis and its Influence on the Respiratory System

Nicole Soucy, MPAS, PA-C*

KEYWORDS

- Allergic rhinitis • Asthma • United airway

KEY POINTS

- Allergic rhinitis is a common condition that affects millions worldwide.
- Allergic rhinitis is an IgE-mediated immune response to various environmental allergens.
- There is evolving evidence demonstrating a link between the nasal mucosa and the airway as a whole.
- Proper evaluation, treatment, and management of allergic rhinitis can benefit the respiratory system.

INTRODUCTION

Colloquially referred to as "hay fever," "cedar fever," or "pollinosis," allergic rhinitis (AR) is a permeating, ubiquitous condition experienced by millions worldwide. Despite its pervasiveness across the globe, its potential consequences on overall health and quality of life are often overlooked. Previously considered to be a localized, bothersome condition without significant consequence, its importance to the entire airway has been better identified in recent years. With our enhanced understanding of the various mechanisms and consequences of AR, our thoughts of AR have shifted from a "disease of the nose" to a multi-faceted condition that affects the respiratory system as a whole."[1] Most importantly, it has been found that rhinitis in general–whether allergic or nonallergic–can impact the development of, severity of, and control of asthma.[1,2] The similarities of the tissues of the upper and lower airway, along with the inflammatory processes involved in both AR and asthma, ultimately leads to a unified response in the face of various environmental allergens.[2] This relationship has been coined by some as "the united airway."

UT Southwestern, Dallas, TX, USA
* 1935 Medical District Drive, F6601.01 Dallas, TX 75235.
E-mail address: nicolesoucypac@gmail.com

Physician Assist Clin 8 (2023) 633–643
https://doi.org/10.1016/j.cpha.2023.06.002
2405-7991/23/© 2023 Elsevier Inc. All rights reserved.

EPIDEMIOLOGY AND RISK FACTORS

As many as 60 million individuals in the United States and 500 million individuals worldwide are affected by allergic rhinitis.[1,3] Within the United States, it is believed to effect more than 40% of children.[3] Additionally, of those with AR, approximately 40% will have comorbid asthma.[4] Other atopic conditions, such as allergic conjunctivitis and atopic dermatitis are other comorbid conditions that often present with AR.[2,5]

It is thought that both environmental and genetics play a role in the development of AR.[1] The biggest risk factor for the development of AR is a family history.[2] Individuals with a family history of AR are up to six times more likely to develop AR than those without a family history.[2] Additional risk factors are outlined in **Box 1**. Conversely, AR is less common in large families and in those who live in rural areas and have exposures to cattle and other livestock.[2]

Rhinitis precedes the development of asthma in approximately 75% of cases, and rhinitis itself is a risk factor for asthma development.[2,4] The majority of asthmatics will have comorbid rhinitis.[1] Both allergic and non-allergic rhinitis can be risk factors for the development of asthma.[1] In fact, it has been demonstrated that worsening rhinitis in individuals with comorbid AR and asthma can lead to worsening asthma symptoms. This can explain why many asthma flares are triggered by viral nasal infections.[1]

Individuals with a family history of AR or asthma are three times more likely to develop asthma.[2] Similar to what is seen in allergic rhinitis, a personal history of atopy prior to the age of 6 is considered to greatly increase the risk of future development of asthma.[2]

Common triggers of AR are outdoor pollens (trees, weeds, grasses), spores from fungi or molds, dander from animals, and droppings from dust mites and cockroaches.[1,3,5] Food allergens are an uncommon cause of AR.[1] Occupational exposures can also impact symptoms of AR and should be considered in adult patients who present with new-onset AR.

DEFINITION

Allergic rhinitis is just one type of rhinitis. AR is an immunoglobulin E (IgE)-mediated immune response to a particular allergen which leads to an inflammatory response within the nasal cavity.[1,3] This inflammatory response produces characteristic symptoms of sneezing, nasal obstruction, rhinorrhea, and nasal pruritus.[1,3] These symptoms can be very burdensome to patients and affect function in daily life.[1,3]

Non-allergic rhinitis (non-IgE mediated rhinitis) can have many different presentations and etiologies. Common types of non-allergic rhinitis include infectious,

---

Box 1
Risk factors for the development of allergic rhinitis

Family history of allergic rhinitis

Serum immunoglobulin E level above >100kU/L before age 6

High socioeconomic status

Urban dwelling

Secondhand smoke exposure

History of positive allergy testing

vasomotor, hormonal, drug-induced, atrophic, and gustatory rhinitis.[3,5,6] To further confound things, it is thought that approximately 35% of patients of AR will also have comorbid non-allergic rhinitis.[5] This is known as "mixed" rhinitis.

Categorizing the severity of AR has evolved as our understanding of the underlying processes has grown. For many years, AR was categorized to be due to either a seasonal, perennial, or occupational trigger.[5] However, given the geographical differences worldwide and that patients are often polysensitized to several allergens, this terminology has become somewhat antiquated. It is now preferable to characterize AR as either "intermittent" or "persistent."[5] Intermittent symptoms are defined as symptoms that occur less than four days a week for less than four weeks while persistent symptoms are present more frequently and for a longer duration.[2] There is more emphasis on classifying AR as either mild, moderate, or severe based on its impact on daily activities, sleep, and the performance at work and school.[2] This categorization is summarized in **Table 1**. The intention of more robust classification of AR is to help guide treatment modalities.

SIGNS/SYMPTOMS

Common symptoms of AR include sneezing, rhinorrhea, congestion, and nasal pruritus.[1–6] Extra-nasal symptoms, such as ocular pruritus and itching of the soft palate, can also be seen.[1–4,6] Uncommon symptoms can include headache, fatigue, and general malaise.[5] Nasal congestion tends to predominate late-stage flares of AR in lieu of typical sneezing and rhinorrhea.[5] These symptoms can be cumbersome and impact sleep as well as performance at work and school.[1,2,4]

Symptoms of asthma include wheezing, tight chest, nocturnal coughing, and dyspnea.[2] Asthma symptoms tend to be worsened by various triggers including illness, exercise, exposure to dust mites and animal dander, changes in temperature, and pollens. Additionally, some medications (such as NSAIDs and β-blockers) can induce asthma symptoms.[2] Exposure to tobacco, whether primary or secondhand smoke, is also a known trigger for asthma.[2]

DIAGNOSIS

Individuals with episodic or persistent nasal congestion, rhinorrhea, nasal pruritus, or sneezing should be evaluated for AR.[3] A careful history should be obtained to identify any possible triggers and risk factors.[3] Understanding if any seasonality to symptoms exists as well as understanding to what degree symptoms impact an individual's daily life–such as work and sleep–can be helpful.[3] Edematous, pale, or purplish nasal turbinates on physical examination are often seen in individuals with AR.[4,5] A linear

Table 1 Classification of rhinitis by frequency and severity of symptoms	
Classification of rhinitits by frequency of symptoms:	
Intermittent symptoms < days per weeks for less than 4 weeks	Persistent symptoms > days per week for greater than 4 weeks
Classification of rhinitits by severity of symptoms	
Mild: No impact on daily activities, sleep, performance at work and school	Moderate/Severe: impact on daily activities, sleep, performance at work and school

crease on the anterior aspect of the nose (also known as an "allergic salute") may also be present.

The most important question to answer is if the rhinitis is allergic or non-allergic in origin.[3] The most common modality of evaluating an individual for aeroallergen sensitivity is either through *in vivo* percutaneous skin prick testing or *in vitro* serum-specific immunoglobulin E testing.[1,2]

Percutaneous skin prick testing has been utilized by practitioners since 1867 and utilizes non-irritating concentrations of a specific allergen extract applied percutaneously to the skin to evaluate for a wheal and flare response.[5,7] Testing is rapid and results are available after approximately 20 minutes.[7] Systemic or life-threatening reactions to percutaneous skin prick testing are extremely rare.[7] This testing requires an individual to withhold antihistamines for several days prior to the testing and is more reliable in children over the age of 2 and adults younger than 65 years old.[7]

While percutaneous skin prick testing is the preferred diagnostic test for the diagnosis of AR, there is also the option of serum-specific immunoglobulin E testing (sIgE). This testing is offered by most commercial laboratories that can measure the degree of sensitivity an individual has to various aeroallergens by measuring the IgE levels associated with each allergen.[5,7] This testing does not require one to withhold antihistamines and is a good alternative to percutaneous skin prick testing when antihistamines cannot be practically or safely discontinued.[5] There is a high false positivity rate to both types of testing and clinical history along with positive testing is necessary to accurately diagnose AR.[1,5]

When the diagnosis of AR is confirmed, it is important to also evaluate for comorbid allergic conjunctivitis, atopic dermatitis, and asthma as these often present in tandem with allergic rhinitis.[1,2]

DIFFERENTIAL

In the absence of positive skin prick testing or sIgE testing, other diagnoses should be considered. Some conditions that can mimic symptoms of AR are the various types of non-allergic rhinitis as well as nasal polyps, foreign bodies, ciliary dysfunction, septal deviation, cerebrospinal fluid leaks, and adenoidal hypertrophy.[2,3]

TREATMENT

At face value, it may seem low yield to focus on the treatment of what is essentially only 0.1% of the body' surface area.[2] However, proper management of AR is necessary to attenuate the severity of asthma in comorbid patients.[2] It has also been found that the treatment of AR can also act as a preventative measure from the development of asthma as well as further aeroallergen sensitivities.[2] Several different treatments for the symptoms AR available include avoidance measures, oral medications, intranasal medications, and systemic therapies. Treatment should be tailored to the individual patient.[1] Each treatment carries its own risks and benefits.

Avoidance Measures

The first treatment in AR should always be the avoidance of offending triggers. Practically speaking, this is not always possible for various reasons.[2] It becomes more difficult to avoid potential triggers in polysensitized individuals. In an idealistic sense, individuals monosensitized to dogs would simply give up their pet dog for a symptom-free life. Realistically, few dog owners would be willing to do this. It is also important to consider psychosocial, emotional, and mental health benefits of pet ownership. Dust mites, molds, and cockroaches are almost impossible to avoid entirely. It is more practical to think of avoidance measures as an important adjunct to pharmaceutical interventions. Some suggested avoidance measures are outlined in **Table 2**.

Intranasal Therapies

In general, intranasal therapies are the first line for the treatment of AR with a primary focus on intranasal corticosteroids.[3] The largest benefit of intranasal therapies is that topical therapy directed at the intended site of action leads to higher concentrations of mediations, faster onset of action, and decreased risks of systemic side effects.[2] The disadvantages of intranasal therapies are that they do not target comorbid atopic conditions such as asthma and atopic dermatitis. These therapies can cause irritation to the nasal mucosa and tend to be dosed more than once daily which can lead to patient noncompliance.[2]

Intranasal corticosteroids

Monotherapy with INCS is generally considered the recommended first-line treatment for AR.[1–4,8] Its effects are multifaceted and regular use can be beneficial in treating nasal pruritus, sneezing, rhinorrhea, and congestion.[2] While primarily used for rhinitis symptom, INCS may also have the benefit on ocular allergy symptoms as well.[3] No specific agent in this class of medication has demonstrated superiority over any other agent.[3]

Clinical response with INCS has been demonstrated to be equal to, if not superior to, oral antihistamines.[2,3] In fact, combination treatment of INCS with an oral antihistamine has not been demonstrated to be superior to INCS therapy alone.[9] Additionally, INCS is preferred over intranasal antihistamines and oral leukotriene inhibitors as a first-line therapy.[10]

Potential side effects can include nasal crusting, epistaxis, and nasal irritation.[2,3] Rarely, septal perforation can occur if used incorrectly.[2,3]

Intranasal antihistamines

Sometimes considered to be "second fiddle" to INCS by clinicians, IAH are still a very powerful treatment in the arsenal to combat AR. While generally less effective than intranasal steroids as a monotherapy, their efficacy is generally considered equal to or superior to second-generation antihistamines.[3] Like INCS, IAH also have the capability to improve ocular allergy symptoms.[1]

Intranasal antihistamines are very safe and work rapidly.[2] Potential side effects include bitter aftertaste, nasal irritation as well as sedation and headache.[3] In some instances, IAH can be used as monotherapy for AR if INCS is not a viable option.[8]

Combined intranasal corticosteroid and intranasal antihistamine

Combinations containing intranasal corticosteroids and intranasal antihistamines (INCS/IAH) are a newer therapy currently available for the treatment of allergic rhinitis in individuals 12 years old and older and has been found to be more effective than monotherapy alone.[8,9] For patients that fail on an INCS monotherapy, it is generally preferred to change a patient to an INCS/IAH combination spray over adding an oral antihistamine.[9] The side effect profile is similar to each of these medications used as monotherapy.[9]

Intranasal chromones (cromolyn)

Intranasal cromolyn is a mast cell stabilizer that can inhibit the release of inflammatory particles involved in AR.[2] It is effective in treating sneezing, rhinorrhea, and nasal

Table 2
Measures and lifestyle modifications to limit aeroallergen exposures

Pollens	Molds	Dust Mites	Cockroach	Animal
Avoid outdoor activity on sunny, windy days with low humidity	Limited avoidance measures available General household hygiene measures, especially in high-moisture areas in the home may be useful	Obtain dust mite impermeable mattress covers and pillowcases as well as HEPA air filtration and vacuum cleaners Lower humidity (dehumidifiers) Limit upholstered furniture Remove carpet in home Wash laundry in hot water (55–60°C)	Consider pest management and traps Keep kitchen clean from food debris	*ONLY demostrated effective measure removal of pet from the home* May be helpful when removal is not an option: Keep pet in a carpet-free room with HEPA air filtration Bathe animal weekly Do not allow pets in bedroom or on high-use furniture

itching.[2] It may have utility as an as-needed treatment to utilize prior to exposure to a known allergen.[8]

While cromolyn is an exceedingly safe treatment for AR with a robust safety profile, its utility is often offset by its limited efficacy in comparison to INCS and oral antihistamines as well as frequent dosing requirements.[1,3] IAH are also preferred over the use of intranasal cromolyn.[10] While a viable option in theory, it is not often utilized in the clinical setting when superior treatments exist.

Intranasal saline
Intranasal saline can be utilized as monotherapy or in conjunction with any other treatment modality for AR. Intranasal saline alone may be attractive in individuals who strongly oppose the use of medications for the treatment of AR. It is generally safe and is effective for chronic rhinorrhea and rhinosinusitis.[1] Intranasal saline is commercially available in various delivery systems such as sprays, aerosols, or lavage. If used correctly, there are minimal side effects, but nasal irritation can occur with overuse.

Intranasal anticholinergics
Given the intrinsic pharmacology of anticholinergic medications, it is no surprise that intranasal anticholinergics are generally effective for persistent rhinorrhea.[1,3,8,10] However, their utility stops with rhinorrhea. They are not very effective for other symptoms of AR, such as nasal congestion, sneezing, nasal obstruction, and nasal pruritus.[2,3] A combination of INCS and intranasal anticholinergic may be more effective in treating rhinorrhea than either agent alone.[3]

Side effects are generally mild and can include dryness of the nares, mouth, and throat as well as nasal irritation, nasal burning, and headache.[2,3] Systemic anticholinergic effects, such as urinary retention, are rare.[2]

Intranasal decongestants
Intranasal decongestants are a double-edged sword in the treatment of AR. Intranasal decongestants work by vasoconstricting the small vessels of the nasal mucosa. It has a rapid onset of action—typically within 10 minutes.[2] Its rapid effects on nasal congestion can be very appealing, but consistent use can lead to significant rebound congestion (also known as rhinitis medicamentosa).[2] It is often used sparingly and with caution among clinicians.[1,3] Intranasal decongestants, while powerful in reducing nasal congestion, does not improve nasal itch, sneezing, or rhinorrhea.[2,3] It can be useful in severe nasal congestion to help facilitate delivery of other intranasal therapies to the targeted areas in the nose that otherwise would be cut off by the congestion, but recommendations are to use for no longer than 5 consecutive days as to prevent rhinitis medicamentosa.[8,10]

Oral Therapies for Allergic Rhinitis

Oral therapies for AR can be useful for those with comorbid conditions beyond AR such as atopic dermatitis or asthma. For instance, some studies have demonstrated that oral second-generation antihistamines may be helpful in the prevention of asthma development in children with dust mite and grass sensitivity.[2] The main disadvantage for oral therapies for AR is that the medications are systemically absorbed with that carry more risk of bothersome systemic side effects.

Oral antihistamines
Oral antihistamines are broken down into two groups: first generation and second generation. First-generation antihistamines are, as their namesake suggests, the first antihistamines that were made available for patient use. They were extremely effective

in treating AR but carried with them significant side effects-namely sedation, CNS depression, and anticholinergic side effects.[2,3] These risks are amplified in elderly individuals.[2] This, compounded with their short half-life and low selectivity, are barriers to their routine use.[2] Their use in the treatment of AR have largely fallen out of favor and their use is generally discouraged.[1,8]

In contrast, newer, second-generation antihistamines now exist which offer a significantly improved side effect profile due to higher selectivity of the H1 receptor, inability to cross the blood–brain barrier, and lack of interaction with cytochrome P450.[2,10] They are less sedative, have a longer half-life, and have a reduced risk of sedative side effects.[2] They are currently recommended over first-generation antihistamines for the treatment of AR in adults and children.[1,3,8,10] They can improve sneezing, rhinorrhea, and nasal pruritus, but they lack efficacy for nasal congestion.[2] They may also be helpful in reducing respiratory symptoms in children.[2] Second generation antihistamines can be used on an as-needed basis but tend to work better when used consistently.[2,3] There is no clinical preference for second-generation antihistamines as there has been no demonstration of superiority with any agent within the group.[3]

Oral leukotriene inhibitors
Agents that act to inhibit leukotrienes can be utilized in AR with comorbid asthma.[3] Leukotriene inhibitors can be helpful for congestion, sneezing, and rhinorrhea.[2] It was previously thought that oral leukotriene inhibitors were effective as monotherapy for the treatment of both conditions, but have more recently fallen out of favor due to emerging evidence that they can present with neuropsychiatric side effects, especially in children.[3,8] For this reason, their use as initial therapy in allergic rhinitis is discouraged, but can be considered when there is failure with a more preferred treatment.[8] The use of INCS and second generation oral antihistamines are still preferred over the use of leukotriene inhibitors as they have demonstrated superior efficacy.[4,9,10]

Oral corticosteroids
In contrast to intranasal corticosteroids—which are generally a staple in the treatment of AR—the use of oral corticosteroids is very limited in the treatment of allergic rhinitis. This is largely due to its significant side effect profile with prolonged use.[3] They are never recommended as first-line treatment.[2,10] That being said, short courses (5–7 days) of oral corticosteroids can be used for severe symptoms of rhinitis, particularly with severe nasal obstruction and anosmia.[2,3,8,10] Parenteral corticosteroids nor long term use of oral corticosteroids are recommended in the treatment of AR.[1,3,8,10]

Oral decongestants
Oral decongestants can be very useful in quickly reducing nasal congestion caused by AR.[2] They are less effective than intranasal decongestants but do not carry the risks of rebound rhinitis medicamentosa with frequent use.[2] Oral decongestants are often found over the counter in combination with oral second-generation antihistamines. While effective in reducing nasal congestion, they carry with them unpleasant side effects such as nasal dryness, palpitations, increased blood pressure, insomnia, and mood side effects (namely irritability).[1–3] These risks are more pronounced in the very young and the elderly.[2,3] Their routine use in the treatment of AR is discouraged but can be a useful adjunct on an as-needed basis in certain patients.[10] Their use is discouraged in individuals with a history of cardiac disease, hyperthyroidism, benign prostatic hypertrophy, and those on β-blockers.[2]

Allergen Immunotherapy

The only disease-modifying treatment available for AR is allergen immunotherapy (AIT).[1,3] Subcutaneous and sublingual routes of AIT are currently available in the United States.[10] Subcutaneous AIT has been around since 1911 and has an excellent track record in its efficacy in reducing AR symptoms.[2] The idea of allergen immunotherapy is to introduce offending aeroallergens to the body to build up tolerance over time by reducing inflammatory mediators released when in contact with the specific allergen.[2] It has been shown to help prevent the development of new aeroallergen sensitivities as well as the development of asthma.[1-3] Additionally, for those with a comorbid diagnosis of asthma, AIT has demonstrated benefit in reducing the severity of asthma symptoms.[3] Long term, sustained benefit from AIT and the reduced need for medications has been well-documented beyond when therapy is completed.[1-3]

It is recommended to pursue AIT for individuals at risk of developing asthma or who already have comorbid, well-controlled asthma and in those with moderate/severe AR who have had failure on other pharmaceutical treatments.[1,8,10]

Potential risks of AIT include the risk of localized swelling, redness, and induration at the site of injection as well as anaphylaxis.[1,2] The risks of severe anaphylaxis are higher in those with uncontrolled asthma and, thus, it is advised to defer AIT in those with uncontrolled asthma.[2] It is known that β-blockers bind to the receptor site of epinephrine-the medication used to treat anaphylaxis—and their use is contraindicated in AIT.[2]

Surgery

While not a cure for AR itself, it bears noting that some surgical procedures may be beneficial in patients with AR who also have structural abnormalities within the nasal cavity as well as those with chronic rhinosinusitis. Septal deviation, turbinate hypertrophy, nasal polyps, and adenoidal hypertrophy can impact nasal congestion and efficacy of the above treatments for AR.[1,3] Surgery is generally considered when all other more conservative treatments have failed. With surgical interventions, as necessary, it may improve the delivery of other treatments for allergic rhinitis and lead to better control of symptoms overall.

DISCUSSION

Allergic rhinitis and the impact it plays on the airway as a whole is finally getting the attention it deserves. Its role in the inflammatory cascade of the respiratory system has grown tremendously over the last twenty years. AR is an extremely common condition, affecting millions worldwide. We now know that having a diagnosis of AR greatly increases the risks of developing asthma, particularly in children. Therefore, it is important to properly treat this condition to alter the natural course and attenuate the risks of developing asthma.

Inflammation that leads to both asthma and allergic rhinitis is caused by an IgE-mediated response to various environmental triggers such as pollens, molds, dust mite, cockroach, animal, and occupational exposures. The first step of confirming AR should be a detailed history followed by environmental allergen testing either with percutaneous skin prick testing or serum-specific IgE testing. Ruling out non-allergic rhinitis or structural abnormalities as a cause for a patient's symptoms is also necessary.

Upon the confirmation of a diagnosis of AR, a multifaceted and individualized approach to the treatment of AR can impact not only the nose but the respiratory system as a whole. Avoidance of triggering allergens should ultimately be the primary treatment in the control of AR, but it is not always feasible or practical. Multiple other treatment modalities such as intranasal, oral, and systemic therapies exist for the treatment of AR, each of them carrying their own potential side effects. Treatments for AR should be chosen carefully based on treatment goals as well as tolerability for the patient.

Ultimately, allergen immunotherapy (AIT) is the only disease-modifying treatment available for AR. Commonly done in an allergy subspeciality office, AIT can not only help reduce further environmental allergen sensitization but can also be preventative for the development of asthma. For those who already have asthma, AIT can improve the control of asthma and lessen its severity as well. Upon the completion of AIT, patients can have sustained unresponsiveness to aeroallergens and require less medications overall.

Comprehensive treatment of the unified airway can have a significant impact in a patient's life. Now that we more fully understand the strong relationship AR and asthma share, we understand that both conditions should be considered in relation to each other. AR should no longer be considered just a bothersome "disease of the nose" but rather a multifaceted condition that impacts the entire airway.

SUMMARY

Allergic rhinitis is hallmarked by sneezing, nasal pruritus, nasal congestion, and rhinorrhea. It affects up to 500 million individuals worldwide. There are multiple different inflammatory processes involved in the development of these symptoms, but an IgE-mediated response to an environmental trigger begins this cascade. Multiple treatment modalities exist with the most preferred options to be avoidance, topical nasal corticosteroids, and allergen immunotherapy.

Allergic rhinitis is a multifaceted condition that should be recognized for its ability to impact more than just the nasal mucosa. It is an extremely common condition that does not always get the attention that it should. Uncontrolled AR not only impacts the quality of life and work performance but also increases the risks of the development of asthma. For those with comorbid AR and asthma, the level of control of AR can directly impact the control of asthma. This unity of the inflammatory processes involved in AR is important to understand to better help patients.

CLINICS CARE POINTS

- Asthma and allergic rhinitis share a significant commonality and often present in tandem
- Proper treatment of allergic rhinitis can impact the development of asthma
- Multiple treatments exist for allergic rhinitis with preference given to avoidance measures, intranasal steroids, and allergen immunotherapy.

DISCLOSURE

The authors have no commercial or financial conflicts of interest. No funding sources have been allotted for the publication of this article.

REFERENCES

1. Bousquet J, Khaltaev N, Cruz AA, et al. Allergic rhinitis and its impact on asthma (ARIA) 2008 update (in collaboration with the World Health Organization, GA(2) LEN and AllerGen). Allergy 2008;63(Suppl 86):8–160.

2. Bousquet J, Van Cauwenberge P, Khaltaev N, Aria Workshop Group; World Health Organization. Allergic rhinitis and its impact on asthma. J Allergy Clin Immunol 2001;108(5 Suppl):S147–334.

3. Wallace DV, Dykewicz MS, Bernstein DI, et al. The diagnosis and management of rhinitis: an updated practice parameter. J Allergy Clin Immunol 2008;122(2 Suppl):S1–84, published correction appears in J Allergy Clin Immunol. 2008 Dec;122(6):1237.

4. Brożek JL, Bousquet J, Agache I, et al. Allergic rhinitis and its impact on asthma (ARIA) guidelines-2016 revision. J Allergy Clin Immunol 2017;140(4):950–8.

5. Quillen DM, Feller DB. Diagnosing rhinitis: allergic vs. nonallergic. Am Fam Physician 2006;73(9):1583–90.

6. Settipane RA, Kaliner MA. Chapter 14: nonallergic rhinitis. Am J Rhinol Allergy 2013;27(Suppl 1):S48–51.

7. Bernstein IL, Li JT, Bernstein DI, et al. Allergy diagnostic testing: an updated practice parameter. Ann Allergy Asthma Immunol 2008;100(3 Suppl 3):S1–148.

8. Dykewicz MS, Wallace DV, Amrol DJ, et al. Rhinitis 2020: a practice parameter update. J Allergy Clin Immunol 2020;146(4):721–67.

9. Dykewicz MS, Wallace DV, Baroody F, et al. Treatment of seasonal allergic rhinitis: an evidence-based focused 2017 guideline update. Ann Allergy Asthma Immunol 2017;119(6):489–511.e41.

10. Brozek JL, Bousquet J, Baena-Cagnani CE, et al. Allergic rhinitis and its impact on asthma (ARIA) guidelines: 2010 revision. J Allergy Clin Immunol 2010;126(3):466–76.

The Asthma Guidline Debate
US vs International Asthma Guidelines - EPR-4 and GINA

Brian Bizik, MS, PA-C

KEYWORDS

- Exhaled nitric oxide (FeNO) • Indoor allergen mitigation • Inhaled corticosteroids
- Long-acting muscarinic antagonists • Allergen immunotherapy
- Bronchial thermoplasty

KEY POINTS

- Two key resources for the management of asthma exist to provide updated treatment guidelines, recommendations to reduce the economic and social burden of asthma and improve the outcome of patients with asthma.
- The Global Initiative for Asthma report (GINA) document is updated annually and is a more comprehensive and complete report that covers diagnosis, treatment options, as well as asthma prevention strategies.
- The National Asthma Education and Prevention Program (NAEPP) meets periodically, most recently reporting in 2020 to address 6 key asthma-related subjects.
- Although both documents can be relevant to daily patient care, GINA will provide guidance on new and emerging topics while the NAEPP updates will aid in the implementation of guideline specifics.

INTRODUCTION
National Asthma Education and Prevention Program Guideline and the Global Initiative for Asthma Report

There are 2 primary asthma resources that can be used by clinicians to guide the evaluation and treatment of asthma: the National Asthma Education and Prevention Program guideline (NAEPP) and the Global Initiative for Asthma report (GINA).

The NAEPP was founded in 1989 through the United States National Heart, Lung, and Blood Institute, Institutes of Health, to develop awareness of the asthma disease state and to help clinicians recognize signs and symptoms of asthma and to ensure effective asthma control within the United States.[1] The first NAEPP was released in 1991 and updated on an as-needed basis (1997, 2002, 2007, 2020). The foundation

Terry Reilly, Health Centers, Idaho State University, 1508 S Gourley Street, Boise, ID 83705, USA
E-mail address: brianbizik@yahoo.com

Physician Assist Clin 8 (2023) 645–652
https://doi.org/10.1016/j.cpha.2023.06.004
2405-7991/23/© 2023 Elsevier Inc. All rights reserved.

of NAEPP reports is based on asking key asthma "questions" to help determine what content should be changed.[2]

GINA was established in 1993 in collaboration with the World Health Organization and the National Heart, Lung, and Blood Institute, National Institutes of Health to determine strategies of asthma care on a global, rather than national, scale. The first GINA report was released in 1995 and subsequently has been updated annually. GINA uses a comprehensive scientific literature review to guide recommendations. Both guidelines are used both in the United States and internationally as guidelines for asthma care.[2]

METHODOLOGY

The NAEPP as well as GINA use recognized asthma researchers and leaders when writing recommendations. Both groups use the Grading of Recommendations Assessment, Development, and Evaluation (GRADE) criteria to assign the relative quality of the evidence presented.

As noted in **Table 1**, the NAEPP's most recent document (2020) used a systematic review of the literature on 6 priority topics through October 2018 conducted by the Agency for Healthcare Research and Quality. The 6 chosen topics were determined based on a needs assessment. Before the 2020 NAEPP (Expert Panel Report 4), nothing had been released since the 2007 NAEPP (Expert Panel Report 3). The GINA asthma workgroup meets twice a year to do an extensive review of published asthma research from the previous 18 months and then publishes their recommendations annually.

Four years before GINA, the NAEPP developed its first Expert Panel Report (EPR): "Guidelines for the Diagnosis and Management of Asthma" in 1991. Following this

Table 1
Differences between global initiative for asthma and national asthma education and prevention program approaches to asthma management

Approach	GINA	NAEPP
Composition of expert panel	Asthma experts from many countries	US-based asthma experts, primary care physicians, ED physicians and input from patients
Target audience	Template for countries to develop their national approach	US based health-care providers and policy makers[1]
Method of literature review	Levels of evidence assigned to management recommendations	GRADE recommendations[3]
Scope	Comprehensive document, regularly reviews current literature	Focused on key topics (6 topics in the most recent focused article)
Guidance on emerging topics	Annually, biologics, COVID-19	Periodically
Access	Online access	Journal of Allergy and Clinical Immunology
Implementation	Global	National

Abbreviations: ED, emergency department; GINA, global initiative for asthma; GRADE, grading of recommendations assessment; NAEPP, national asthma education and prevention program.
Szefler SJ. Update on the NAEPPCC Asthma Guidelines: The wait is over, or is it? J Allergy Clin Immunol. 2020;146(6):1275–1280.

initial report, there was a complete guideline revision, EPR-2 published in 1997. The last complete revision, EPR-3 was published in 2003. Most recently, in 2020, the National Asthma Education and Prevention Program Coordinating Committee released its focused update on 6 key subjects of fraction of exhaled nitric oxide (FeNO), indoor allergen mitigation, inhaled corticosteroids, long-acting muscarinic antagonists (LAMAs), allergen immunotherapy, and bronchial thermoplasty (BT).[4]

We will examine the similarities and differences in these 6 areas.

Fractional Exhaled Nitric Oxide

FeNO is measured in the exhaled breath of patients and has been used as a noninvasive way to assess and monitor airway inflammation. It was found that FeNO levels decreased in patients in response to treatment with corticosteroids, thus possibly providing information about which treatments were most likely to be helpful for a given patient.[5] FeNO levels have also been used to assess and monitor airway inflammation in asthma. Higher levels of FENO (>50 ppb in adults and >35 ppb in children aged 5–12 years) in nonsmokers has been found to be associated with eosinophilic airway inflammation.

Concerning the use of FeNO, both GINA and the NAEPP generally support the use of FeNO as an adjunct to assist in determining levels of airway inflammation.[5] When FeNO is used to guide therapeutic decisions in children, there was a significant decrease in asthma exacerbations compared with management based on symptoms alone. The GINA guidelines consider there to be strong evidence supporting the use of FeNO while the most recent NAEPP article stated that FeNO, in isolation, is not useful for an asthma diagnosis in patients aged older than 5 years.[6] Also noting that FeNO should not be used in young children to predict the future development of asthma.[6] Both groups do support the use of FeNO as an adjunct to determine the need for increasing therapy or adding anti-inflammatory therapy.

Indoor Allergen Mitigation

A central feature of the management of indoor asthma triggers when the asthma patient has a known sensitivity to a specific allergen. Indoor allergen exposure can increase both asthma and other allergic symptoms. Allergens in the indoor environment include dust mites, pet dander, and molds.[7] Allergen reduction interventions decrease exposure to the known allergen and can be single intervention (an attempt to reduce a single-targeted allergen) or a multifactor intervention (targeting several possible allergens).[7] Both the GINA and the NAEPP recommendations support the use of impermeable bedding encasements as a part of a multicomponent allergen reduction plan for those with known or suspected allergy to dust mite.[4] For the reduction or removal of indoor molds GINA has a level A recommendation while the NAEPP provides a lower certainty of the evidence.

Overall, the NAEPP recommends a multicomponent allergen reduction plan for those patients with asthma with known indoor allergen sensitivity. This recommendation also applies to those with known pest sensitization.[8] GINA does not recommend allergen avoidance as a general strategy for those without documented sensitivity to indoor allergens and reports that there is limited evidence of clinical benefit in a single-component strategy. Similar to the NAEPP, the current GINA recommendation does support a trial of indoor mitigation in those with known sensitization only when it is part of a comprehensive mitigation strategy.[8]

Inhaled corticosteroid use

Both GINA and NAEPP divide recommendations for inhaled corticosteroid use into groups based on age. We will compare various age groups in this next section.

The initial group for guideline recommendations is children aged 5 years and younger in the GINA article and children aged 0 to 4 years in the NAEPP report.[4] GINA classifies these children as Step 1 when the reported symptoms are a few virally mediated wheezing episodes with minimal symptoms between flares. Recommendations for children in Step 1 are for no daily controller and as needed, short-acting beta-2 agonist (SABA).[9] When symptoms have increased and there are wheezing episodes more than 3 times a year, GINA classifies patients as Step 2 with a preferred controller therapy for inhaled low-dose inhaled corticosteroid for a period of 3 months.[9]

The NEAPP recommendations for children aged 0 to 4 years, with recurrent wheezing episodes, NAEPP classifies them as Step 1 with intermittent asthma. For this group, the preferred treatment is a short course of daily high-dose inhaled corticosteroid for 7 to 10 days and as needed SABA at the start of a respiratory tract infection or wheezing/cough exacerbation.[10,11]

The data for the use of periodic therapy, in this case inhaled corticosteroids for young children, can be found in studies cited by both GINA and the NAEPP. Key studies include Ducharme and colleagues where it was found that starting high-dose fluticasone early in the course of a respiratory tract infection reduced symptom duration and severity, decreased days of SABA use, reduced the need for additional oral steroid therapy, and asthma's negative effect on quality of life.[9] Another key study, Kaiser and colleagues, using a meta-analysis of evidence found high-dose intermittent inhaled corticosteroid (ICS) taken during 7 to 10 days at the first indication of a respiratory infection had a 35% risk reduction in severe asthma exacerbations and decreased emergency room visits and overall need for inpatient care.[9]

For children that are older, between the ages of 5 and 11 years, the NAEPP suggests that daily low-dose ICS is the preferred treatment of choice for mild persistent asthma and notes this group in Step 2. For adolescents (aged 12 years and older) as well as adults, the NAEPP has 2 preferred treatment choices for mild persistent asthma. One option is daily low-dose ICS with as-needed SABA. The second option is as-needed use ICS and SABA, to be taken at the same time. This would start at the first sign of asthma symptoms. These US-based guidelines to recommend that patients who have a low perception of symptoms are more likely to have severe exacerbations and should not use intermittent maintenance therapy. For these patients, daily maintenance therapy is recommended.[12]

The GINA guidelines for patients aged 6 to 11 years recommend as-needed intermittent low-dose ICS to be taken whenever SABA is taken for Step 1. For 12 years and older, the preferred treatment is a combination of as-needed inhaled ICS with formoterol for Steps 1 and 2 with the alternative treatment option being ICS whenever SABA is taken.[4] One noted difference is how the 2 groups classify asthma severity. NAEPP continues to classify asthma as intermittent and mild, moderate, and severe persistent based on symptom frequency. GINA also includes mild, moderate, and severe asthma severity classifications; however, the emphasis in the GINA guidelines is that asthma severity should be based on treatment required to control the patients symptoms as well as exacerbations rather than using symptom frequency as the primary factor.[13] This distinction is quite important because while the US-based recommendations in the NAEPP suggest treatment with SABA alone in patients aged 5 to 11 years in Step 1, and daily preventative ICS and intermittent SABA in step 2 (mild persistent asthma), GINA suggests treating mild intermittent and mild persistent asthma in patients aged 12 years and older with the same regiment of only using ICS-formoterol as needed for symptom relief.[14]

Long-acting muscarinic antagonist

LAMA medications provide bronchodilation through inhibition of the muscarinic receptors on the bronchioles causing relaxation of the smooth muscle. LAMAs work by blocking acetylcholine, which prevents vagal nerve-induced bronchoconstriction and reduces overall mucus secretions.[15] There are key differences in the 2 guidelines with respect to LAMA use. NAEPP conditionally recommends against adding a (LAMA) to inhaled steroid therapy when compared with inhaled corticosteroid - long-acting beta-agonist (ICS-LABA) in individuals aged 12 years and older with uncontrolled asthma. These guidelines note that the LABA benefit was more favorable than the addition of a LAMA medication. NAEPP did conditionally recommend adding a LAMA to ICS in patients aged older than 12 years if they were not able to tolerate LABA and were not well controlled on ICS alone.[16] GINA recommendations differ considerably. For patients aged 12 years and older, GINA notes that a LAMA may be considered but not to be used in children aged 6 to 11 years.[16] LAMAs can be used as a triple combination inhaler therapy for individuals aged older than 18 years if asthma is poorly controlled and on at least medium-to high-dose ICS-LABA. GINA does not specifically address whether LABAs are preferred to add on therapy over LAMAs when someone is not controlled with asthma alone.[17] The guidelines do agree that LAMAs should not be added to any patients without first starting with an inhaled corticosteroid.

Allergy immunotherapy

Many patients with asthma have other atopic conditions. This can include allergic rhinitis. This is especially true of patients with allergic asthma. Allergic asthma is a type of asthma frequently encountered by practitioners and is defined as having an increase in asthma symptoms after exposure to an allergen or during an allergy season.[18] Allergy immunotherapy can be an important part of the overall treatment of patients with allergic asthma. This therapy incorporates incremental high-dose exposure to a known allergen over time, reducing immunoglobulin E–mediated allergic clinical response.[18]

Immunotherapy, or allergy shots, is often administered subcutaneously but can also be administered sublingually.[19] NAEPP provides a conditional recommendation for the use of subcutaneous allergen immunotherapy as an adjunct therapy for children aged older than 5 years who have demonstrated allergic sensitization or worsening asthma symptoms in mild-to-moderate allergic asthma.[19] NAEPP guidelines do not however support the use of sublingual immunotherapy for the treatment of asthma. GINA recommends allergen-specific immunotherapy as a treatment option if the allergen plays a role in the patient's allergic rhinitis or other allergic conditions.[20]

Bronchial thermoplasty

BT was approved by the US Food and Drug Administration in 2010 and has been used successfully since.[21] BT has been shown to be a safe procedure and is indicated for the treatment of severe persistent asthma that is not controlled with high-dose inhaled corticosteroids and LABA inhaler therapy.[21] This lung treatment delivers local radiofrequency energy to the large airways causing airway remodeling by reducing airway smooth muscle. The composition of the extracellular milieu is modulated as well.[22] This procedure decreases hypertrophied airway smooth muscle that contributes to airway hyperreactivity in severe asthmatics. NAEPP does not recommended bronchial thermoplasty as a treatment option for persistent asthma because the small benefit does not outweigh the risks, which include atelectasis and infection.[23] GINA similarly

---

Box 1
Six key questions of the national asthma education and prevention program expert panel working group[4]

Use of FeNO

Indoor allergen mitigation

Inhaled corticosteroids

Long-acting muscarinic antagonists

Allergen immunotherapy

Bronchial thermoplasty

---

states that bronchial thermoplasty is a potential treatment option for adults whose asthma is uncontrolled despite the regular use of optimal asthma therapy.[23]

Coronavirus disease 2019, asthma, and guideline recommendations

The worldwide pandemic of CORONAVIRUS disease 2019 (COVID-19) has affected patients with asthma of all severities. Patients with COVID-19 presented with a wide variety of symptoms that often included a dry cough, fever, fatigue, body aches, loss of taste and smell, as well as shortness of breath.[4] More severe patients progressed to pneumonia and even respiratory failure. Respiratory viruses such as COVID-19 are a common trigger for asthma and can lead to asthma exacerbations, emergency visits, and hospitalizations. During the past 2 years of COVID-19 infection and disease surveillance, it was found that individuals with well-controlled mild-to-moderate asthma have no increased risk of acquiring COVID-19 or experiencing more severe symptoms from COVID-19.[24] The increased risk of COVID-19-related hospitalizations and mortality with asthma was largely associated with age and other coexisting comorbidities such as heart disease and diabetes. The most recent NAEPP guidelines did not address asthma management in the face of COVID-19.[2] GINA recommendations include the importance that individuals with asthma to have a written asthma action plan and encourages them to continue taking medications, particularly any inhaled corticosteroids. GINA also recommends receiving the COVID-19 vaccine.[1]

SUMMARY—GUIDELINE IMPLEMENTATION

Both the NAEPP and GINA guidelines are designed to provide evidence-based reports that can be incorporated into the asthma practice of both the general practitioner and the asthma specialist.[4] The various approaches are outlined below in **Box 1**. GINA specifically provides a step-by-step approach designed to be used by health-care practitioners at all levels.[1] GINA provides its recommendations with the assessment of the individual needs by evaluating resources as well as the cultural and economic environment and does so on an annual basis. Because of this, the GINA published guidelines are often the first, and most common, guideline used worldwide.[25] The NAEPP recommendations are question based. Each update seeking to review specific questions often provides a more in-depth look at specific asthma topics. The frequency of NAEPP reporting is irregular and difficult to predict.

For those that diagnose and treat asthma, reviewing both the NAEPP and GINA recommendations should be done on a regular basis and the data within incorporated into asthma therapy. Although there are differences in the 2 reports, the increased therapeutic options for health-care practitioners will aid in providing individual care for patients with asthma.

CLINICS CARE POINTS

- Asthma guidelines can help guide medical decision-making for the diagnosis and treatment of asthma.
- Two well-recognized asthma guidelines exist—the US NAEPP guidelines, which are updated periodically (last in 2020), and the GINA, which are updated annually or semiannually.
- The most recent US guidelines focused on 6 key asthma questions as well as an update on treatment progression.
- GINA guidelines are a comprehensive review of asthma literature and provide a stepwise approach to diagnosis and asthma care.
- Both guidelines recommend step up therapy because asthma symptoms increase and stress asthma symptom control over rescue therapy.

DISCLOSURE

The author has nothing to disclose.

REFERENCES

1. Global Initiative for Asthma. Global strategy for asthma management and prevention. 2021. Available from: www.ginasthma.org. Accessed December 12, 2022. This is a comprehensive document that is updated annually with review and best recommendation strategy for national guideline development.
2. Szefler SJ. Update on the NAEPPCC Asthma Guidelines: the wait is over, or is it? J Allergy Clin Immunol 2020;146:1275–80. This is an outstanding rostrum comparing the different approaches to asthma management between GINA and the NAEPP.
3. GRADE. The Grading of Recommendations Assessment, Development and Evaluation Working Group. Available at: https://www.gradeworkinggroup. org/. Accessed December 12, 2022.
4. Cloutier M, Baptist A, Blake K, et al. Expert Panel Working Group of the National Heart, Lung, and Blood Institute (NHLBI) administered and coordinated National Asthma Education and Prevention Program Coordinating Committee (NAEPPCC). 2020 focused updates to the asthma management guidelines: a report from the National Asthma Education and Prevention Program Coordinating Committee Expert Panel Working Group. J Allergy Clin Immunol 2020;146:1217–70. The United States National Guidelines focused updates on six key subjects provides best practice recommendations for asthma.
5. Silkoff PE, McClean P, Spino M, et al. Dose– response relationship and reproducibility of the fall in exhaled nitric oxide after inhaled beclomethasone dipropionate therapy in asthma patients. Chest 2001;119:1322–8.
6. Wang Z, Pianosi P, Keogh K, et al. The clinical utility of fractional exhaled nitric oxide (FeNO) in asthma management [Internet]. Rockville (MD): Agency for Healthcare Research and Quality (US); 2017. Dec. Report No.: 17(1 8)- EHCO30-EF.
7. Leas BF, D'Anci KE, Apter AJ, et al. Effectiveness of indoor allergen reduction in asthma management: a systematic review. J Allergy Clin Immunol 2018;141:1854–69.
8. Matsui EC, Peng RD. 2020 Updated Asthma Guidelines: indoor allergen reduction. J Allergy Clin Immunol 2020;146:1283–5.

9. Kaiser SV, Huynh T, Bacharier LB, et al. Preventing exacerbations in preschoolers with recurrent wheeze: a meta-analysis. Pediatrics 2016;137:e20154496.

10. Bacharier LB, Phillips BR, Zeiger RS, et al. Episodic use of an inhaled corticosteroid or leukotriene receptor antagonist in preschool children with moderate-to-severe intermittent wheezing. J Allergy Clin Immunol 2008;122:1127–35.

11. Stokes JR, Bacharier LB. Prevention and treatment of recurrent viral-induced wheezing in the preschool child. Ann Allergy Asthma Immunol 2020;125: 156–62. This review is an excellent summary of evidence in the treatment of viral-induced wheezing in young children.

12. Generoso A, Tuong L-A, Oppenheimer J. Treatment strategies for the yellow zone. Ann Allergy Asthma Immunol 2019;123:345–51.

13. Kew KM, Quinn M, Quon BS, et al. Increased versus stable doses of inhaled corticosteroids for exacerbations of chronic asthma in adults and children. Cochrane Database Syst Rev 2016;6:CD007524.

14. Oborne J, Mortimer K, Hubbard RB, et al. Quadrupling the dose of inhaled corticosteroid to prevent asthma exacerbations: a randomized, double-blind, placebo-controlled, parallel-group clinical trial. Am J Respir Crit Care Med 2009; 180:598–602.

15. Jorup C, Lythgoe D, Bisgaard H. Budesonide/formoterol maintenance and reliever therapy in adolescent patients with asthma. Eur Respir J 2018;51:1701688.

16. O'Byrne PM, Bisgaard H, Godard PP, et al. Budesonide/formoterol combination therapy as both maintenance and reliever medication in asthma. Am J Respir Crit Care Med 2005;171:129–36.

17. Reddel HK, FitzGerald JM, Bateman ED, et al. GINA 2019: a fundamental change in asthma management: treatment of asthma with short-acting bronchodilators alone is no longer recommended for adults and adolescents. Eur Respir J 2019;53:1901046.

18. Lin SY, Azar A, Suarez-Cuervo C, et al. The role of immunotherapy in the treatment of asthma [Internet]. Rockville (MD): Agency for Healthcare Research and Quality (US); 2018. Mar. Report No.: 17(18)-EHC029- EF.

19. Abramson MJ, Puy RM, Weiner JM. Injection allergen immunotherapy for asthma. Cochrane Database Syst Rev 2010;8:CD001186.

20. Nelson HS. 2020 Updated Asthma Guidelines: allergen immunotherapy. J Allergy Clin Immunol 2020;146:1286–7. This excellent editorial reviews the NAEPPCC Asthma Guidelines 2020 topic on allergen immunotherapy.

21. Chaudhuri R, Rubin A, Sumino K, et al. Safety and effectiveness of bronchial thermoplasty after 10 years in patients with persistent asthma: a follow-up of three randomized controlled trials. Lancet Respir Med 2021;9:457–66.

22. Tan LD, Yoneda KY, Louie S, et al. Bronchial thermoplasty: a decade of experience: state of the art. J Allergy Clin Immunol Pract 2019;7:71–80.

23. Chupp G, Laviolette M, Cohn L. Long-term outcomes of bronchial thermoplasty in subjects with severe asthma: a comparison of 3-year follow-up results from two prospective multicentre studies. Eur Respir J 2017;50:1750017.

24. Organization WH. WHO Director-General's opening remarks at the Mission briefing on COVID-19-12 March 2020. Available at: https://www.who.int/dg/speeches/detail/who-director-general-s-opening-remarks-at-the-missionbriefing-on-covid-19. Accessed December 12, 2022.

25. Israel E. Implementing the guidelines: what do you do when the rubber hits the road? J Allergy Clin Immunol 2020;146:1271–4.

Pediatric Asthma and Allergy

Kimberly Poarch, MPAS, PA-C

KEYWORDS

- Asthma • Pediatric • Allergy • Atopy • Spirometry • Asthma control

KEY POINTS

- Asthma is the most common chronic disease in pediatric populations.
- Asthma is often associated with other forms of atopy, including allergic rhinitis, atopic dermatitis, and food allergies.
- Tools are available to predict the development of asthma in young children.
- Proper asthma treatment includes prevention or reversal of bronchoconstriction and prevention or treatment of inflammation.
- Lifestyle modifications can prevent the escalation of asthma.

BACKGROUND

Asthma is a common respiratory disease, characterized by chronic inflammation and hyperreactivity in the airway. Asthma affects children but is difficult to diagnose accurately in the younger population. Efforts have been made to create useful and accurate tools to predict the development of asthma in younger children. Using these tools effectively can help to prevent symptom onset and initiate proper treatment in a timelier manner, hopefully preventing significant morbidity and severity of symptoms. Ultimately, effective trigger avoidance measures, proper pharmacologic therapy, allergen immunotherapy in appropriate patients, and close medical follow-up with the proper use of functional tools will benefit pediatric patients with asthma.

INTRODUCTION

Asthma is the most common disease in pediatric populations and is estimated to affect 7 million children in the United States.[1] An estimated $81 million is the financial burden of asthma in the United States each year, and children miss more than 14 million school days annually due to asthma.[2–4] Development of asthma is multifactorial and influenced by both inherited and external variables. Diagnosis of asthma in children is challenging, due to the variable nature of the disease and symptoms, and because lung function tests are difficult to perform in children and are less specific

Allergy & Asthma Specialists, 10100 North Central Expressway, Suite 100, Dallas, TX 75231, USA
E-mail address: poarchpac@allergyspecialists.us

Physician Assist Clin 8 (2023) 653–662
https://doi.org/10.1016/j.cpha.2023.06.005
2405-7991/23/© 2023 Elsevier Inc. All rights reserved.

and sensitive than in adults. When providing medical care to pediatric patients, we may use tools to help predict which patients are most at risk of developing asthma. Patients identified to be at higher risk of developing asthma may benefit from more aggressive environmental exposure prevention measures, earlier pharmaceutical interventions, and referral to an allergy specialist for evaluation and treatment.

RISK FACTORS OF ASTHMA IN PEDIATRIC PATIENTS

The development of asthma is influenced by multiple factors including genetics, environmental exposures, psychosocial disparities, and other variables. Recognizing these factors can clue us into the need for risk assessment of future asthma development. Gaining control of the things that can be modified is an important step in the prevention and treatment of this significant disease. **Box 1** lists common risk factors for childhood asthma.[5]

PREDICTION TOOLS OF ASTHMA DEVELOPMENT

The presence of multiple episodes of wheezing is a predictor of future asthma. Various tools have been developed to help predict the likelihood of developing childhood asthma, and many include the occurrence of early childhood wheezing episodes as a factor. Two tools that have been studied and used are the Modified Asthma Predictive Index (mAPI) and the Pediatric Asthma Risk Score (PARS).

Modified Asthma Predictive Index

The mAPI was developed to predict the development of asthma more accurately in children compared with the Asthma Predictive Index (API), which had fewer criteria and was less able to accurately predict mild-to-moderate asthma. By adding more criteria points, the mAPI was proven superior to the API at predicting future asthma if positive.

A positive mAPI requires at least 4 wheezing episodes plus 1 major or 2 minor criteria during the first 3 years of life.

Major criteria in the Modified Asthma Predictive Index

- Confirmed diagnosis of asthma in a parent
- Confirmed diagnosis of atopic dermatitis
- Allergic sensitization (IgE) to at least one aeroallergen as confirmed by skin prick testing or serum-specific immunoglobulin E testing (sIgE)

Box 1
Common risk factors for asthma[5]

Family history of atopy (allergies, asthma, and eczema)

Second-hand smoke exposure before or after birth

Low birth weight

Allergies

Eczema

Early or frequent respiratory infections

Growing up in a low income, urban environment

Minor criteria in the Modified Asthma Predictive Index

- Allergic sensitization (IgE) to food allergen as confirmed by skin prick testing or sIgE
- Wheezing unrelated to colds
- Peripheral Eosinophilia

A positive mAPI indicates a significant increase in the probability of asthma by the age of 11 years, especially in higher-risk patients. Unfortunately, a negative mAPI does not indicate a meaningful probability of a patient not developing asthma in the future.[6]

Pediatric asthma risk score

To identify additional pediatric patients at risk of developing asthma who did not meet the criteria through the API, the PARS tool was developed as another option to the mAPI. By adding more variables to consider, PARS captures the prediction of more mild-to-moderate asthma by the age of 7 years than API or mAPI does. It also provides a low–moderate–high risk range rather than a positive or negative result when applied.

Criteria points used in the PARS:

- Parental asthma (2 points)
- Atopic dermatitis before age 3 years (2 points)
- Wheezing unrelated to colds (3 points)
- Wheezing before age 3 years (3 points)
- African-American Race (2 points)
- Positive IgE sensitization to 2 or more aero or food allergens (2 points)[1,7]

A web-based PARS calculator as well as links to the PARS mobile application are available at https://pars.research.cchmc.org/ through the Cincinnati Children's Hospital Medical Center (**Fig. 1**).[8]

Ultimately, no tool is perfectly accurate to predict the development of asthma. The usefulness of tools may be limited by many variables, including the parent's accurate recall of past events, a patient's access to medical care, access to accurate allergy testing, and bias to only screen high-risk patients. Not all tools have been studied and verified in large, diverse populations, so additional study is always needed. Also, there is no one tool that is recommended across the board. Keeping all these in mind, an awareness of available tools, and the utilization of appropriate tools in your particular practice will help to identify patients who may benefit from early intervention.[7]

DIAGNOSING ASTHMA

Symptoms of asthma illustrate the inflammation and obstruction in the airway, and may include

- Wheezing
- Dry cough
- Chest tightness
- Chest congestion
- Fatigue
- Chronic cough
- Dyspnea
- Clear or white sputum production
- Labored breathing
- Chest pain

Pediatric Asthma Risk Score (PARS) Sheet

	Possible Scores		Child's Score
	No	Yes	
1. Parental Asthma	0	2	
2. Eczema before age 3 y	0	2	
3. Wheezing apart from colds	0	3	
4. Wheezing before age 3 y	0	3	
5. African-American Race	0	2	
6. SPT positive to ≥ 2 aero and/or food allergens	0	2	
Child's PARS (add lines 1-6 above):			

Patient Score Interpretation

Score	Risk of Asthma by age 7 years		Interpretation
0	3%		Children with these scores have a 1 in 33 [score of 0] to a 1 in 9 [score of 4] risk of developing asthma by age 7 y
2	6%	LOW RISK	
3	8%		
4	11%		
5	15%	MODERATE RISK	Children with these scores have a 1 in 7 risk [Score of 5] to a 1 in 3 [Score of 8] risk of developing asthma by age 7 y
6	19%		
7	25%		
8	32%		
9	40%	HIGH RISK	Children with these scores have a 2 in 5 [Score of 9] to a 4 in 5 [Score of 14] risk of developing asthma by age 7 y
10	49%		
11	58%		
12	66%		
14	79%		

Fig. 1. PARS sheet.[8] (*From* Pediatric Asthma Risk Score. Available at https://pars.research.cchmc.org/. Accessed November 30, 2022.)

These symptoms are frequently episodic and intermittent, with potential for complete resolution between exacerbations. Symptoms may be provoked with many triggers, including exercise, viral respiratory illness, exposure to irritants or allergens, cold air, laughter, and during nocturnal hours. Recognizing the symptoms, triggers, and repeated episodes of symptom occurrence by the medical provider, parents, and eventually by the patient is key to establishing a diagnosis of asthma and treating appropriately. When symptoms have been noted, a detailed history should be obtained. Symptom triggers, family and patient history of allergies, and response to previous treatment regimen are valuable details.

The examination of a patient suspected to have asthma may vary by age and severity of symptoms. Although some patients may have coughing and wheezing, especially on exhalation, others may have none. Infants and toddlers may be listless or have less interest in feeding. A severely affected patient may have an increased respiratory rate and will be using accessory muscles for inspiration. Patients often have signs of atopy, such as allergic rhinitis or allergic conjunctivitis, and eczema. For patients 5 years and older, breathing tests may be done to measure for obstruction and inflammation, including spirometry and exhaled nitric oxide (FeNO). Although demonstrating a greater than or equal to 12% improvement in forced expiratory volume in the first second (FEV1) measurements by spirometry after bronchodilator administration is specific for asthma diagnosis, it can be difficult for children to perform this test consistently. FeNO can help identify patients with chronic inflammation, but can be elevated with other conditions, and is probably most helpful in monitoring how a patient with asthma responds to asthma treatment. Other tests that contribute to the diagnosis of asthma are specific IgE allergen testing by serum or skin prick as well as serum total IgE and absolute eosinophil levels that may be best performed by an asthma specialist such as a PA or NP who specializes in allergy or asthma or a board-certified allergist.[9]

Often the diagnosis of asthma is made clinically based on the signs, symptoms, pattern of episodes, and positive response to bronchodilator and anti-inflammatory medications that will be discussed below. Although a definitive diagnosis is made with post bronchodilator response as measured by spirometry, it is not required for making the diagnosis of pediatric asthma and should not delay the initiation of appropriate treatment.

MANAGEMENT OF ASTHMA

The goals of the treatment of asthma are

- To reduce acute symptoms
- Prevent exacerbations
- Reduce risk of remodeling of airways

By meeting these goals, patients will have better symptom control, avoid absences in school and work, be able to perform activities as desired, and minimize risk of severe disease progression.

CATEGORIZATION OF CURRENT ASTHMA STATE

Once a patient has been officially diagnosed with asthma and before initiating treatment, an assessment of the asthma severity should be performed. Severity can be determined by how often symptoms occur (intermittent vs persistent), and how greatly the symptoms are affecting the patient. Assessments should also be done at future visits, both at routine visits and during visits when the patient is having asthma symptoms.[10]

Standardized tools, such as the Childhood ACT (Asthma Control Test), are scored by the parent and patient based on criteria centered around the frequency and timing of symptoms and ability to participate in activities, all within the previous 4 week period. The ACT simply assesses if a patient's asthma is controlled or uncontrolled based on the cumulative score. When ACT is used over time, it can be helpful to view how controlled a patient is in different seasons or ages. The ACT questions can also educate the patient and parents about the signs of worsening asthma control (Fig. 2).[11,12]

Other standardized questionnaires are available and may be used to gather information for patients of specific age groups and those performing specific activities. Many other questionnaires exist, including

- ACT (for 12 y/o and older).
- Asthma Control Questionnaire
- Pediatric Asthma Control and Communication Instrument

Enter Name _____   Today's Date: _____

Enter Address _____   Patient's Name: _____

Enter City/State/Zip _____

Childhood Asthma Control Test for children 4 to 11 years.

This test will provide a score that may help the doctor determine if your child's asthma treatment plan is working or if it might be time for a change.

How to take the Childhood Asthma Control Test

Step 1 Let your child respond to the first four questions (1 to 4). If your child needs help reading or understanding the question, you may help, but let your child select the response. Complete the remaining three questions (5 to 7) on your own and without letting your child's response influence your answers. There are no right or wrong answers.

Step 2 Write the number of each answer in the score box provided.

Step 3 Add up each score box for the total.

Step 4 Take the test to the doctor to talk about your child's total score.

19 or less If your child's score is 19 or less, it may be a sign that your child's asthma is not controlled as well as it could be. Bring this test to the doctor to talk about the results.

Have your child complete these questions.

1. How is your asthma today?

| 0 Very bad | 1 Bad | 2 Good | 3 Very good | SCORE |

2. How much of a problem is your asthma when you run, exercise or play sports?

| 0 It's a big problem, I can't do what I want to do. | 1 It's a problem and I don't like it. | 2 It's a little problem but it's okay. | 3 It's not a problem. |

3. Do you cough because of your asthma?

| 0 Yes, all of the time. | 1 Yes, most of the time. | 2 Yes, some of the time. | 3 No, none of the time. |

4. Do you wake up during the night because of your asthma?

| 0 Yes, all of the time. | 1 Yes, most of the time. | 2 Yes, some of the time. | 3 No, none of the time. |

Please complete the following questions on your own.

5. During the last 4 weeks, how many days did your child have any daytime asthma symptoms?

| 5 Not at all | 4 1-3 days | 3 4-10 days | 2 11-18 days | 1 19-24 days | 0 Everyday |

6. During the last 4 weeks, how many days did your child wheeze during the day because of asthma?

| 5 Not at all | 4 1-3 days | 3 4-10 days | 2 11-18 days | 1 19-24 days | 0 Everyday |

7. During the last 4 weeks, how many days did your child wake up during the night because of asthma?

| 5 Not at all | 4 1-3 days | 3 4-10 days | 2 11-18 days | 1 19-24 days | 0 Everyday |

TOTAL

Fig. 2. Childhood asthma control test.[12] (*From* Childhood Asthma Control Test https://www.nationaljewish.org/NJH/media/pdf/pdf-Childhood_ACT.pdf, Accessed January 22, 2023.)

- Asthma APGAR (Activities, Persistent Triggers, Asthma medications, and Response to therapy)

Whichever tool is chosen, consistent use of said tool will offer a snapshot of current asthma state, an assessment of risk for future symptoms, and a marker of response to treatment when used over longer periods of time.

Spirometry can also help categorize the severity of asthma and should be performed to assess the current state of lung function and the response to therapy. FENO measurements may supplement these assessments as well.[11]

PHARMACOLOGIC THERAPY

After determining the frequency and severity of asthma, all asthma patients must be considered for pharmaceutical therapy. Treatments are recommended in a stepwise manner, so that patients with severe or worsening symptoms may be stepped up in therapy, whereas patients who remain well controlled may be considered for a step down in therapy. The National Asthma Education and Prevention Program (NAEPP) provides treatment guidelines based on the age of the patient. Here is an example for patients aged 5 to 11 years old (**Fig. 3**).[13]

The Global Initiative for Asthma offers a *Global Strategy for Asthma Management and Prevention* from an international panel of experts in pulmonary medicine. This set of guidelines also recommends a stepwise approach to selecting appropriate treatment of patients. A personal use download is available at https://ginasthma.org/gina-reports/.[14]

Medication choices recommended in guidelines may be individualized to each patient, considering various factors including formulation, cost, preference, availability, dosing schedule, and tolerance. Categories of preferred medications in pediatric asthma patients include

- SABA: inhaled short-acting β_2 agonist; relieves bronchoconstriction acutely
- ICS: inhaled corticosteroid; prevents inflammation
- LABA: inhaled long-acting β_2 agonist; relieves bronchoconstriction more than 12 to 24 hours
- OCS: oral systemic corticosteroids; decreases and prevents inflammation

Alternative treatment medication options include

- LTRA: leukotriene receptor antagonist; prevents late phase inflammation
- Cromolyn: prevents mast cell degranulation
- Theophylline: bronchodilator
- LAMA: inhaled long-acting muscarinic antagonist; long-acting bronchodilator

Adjunct treatments under the care of an asthma or allergy specialist include

- SCIT: subcutaneous immunotherapy; gradually builds tolerance to exposure of allergens
- Biologic therapy: specific antibody or cell targeted treatment to reduce chronic inflammation[15]

Depending on the step level an asthma patient is determined to currently be, a combination of the medication types listed above may be needed to gain control of symptoms and prevent future exacerbations. Potential side effects should be discussed with patients as well. Each medication type addresses a different component of asthma symptomatology, and when used in conjunction may provide more complete control.[13]

PATIENT EDUCATION AND LIFESTYLE MODIFICATIONS

Patients and their parents are vital partners in the control of asthma, and must be educated about the disease process, recognition of symptoms, medications

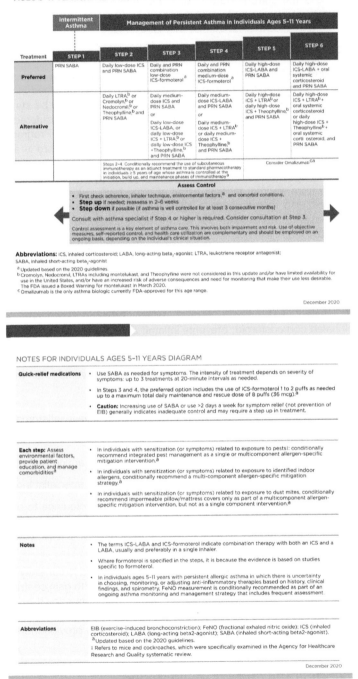

Fig. 3. NAEPP age 5 to 11 years: stepwise approach for management of asthma.[13] (*From 2020 Focused Updates to the Asthma Management Guidelines: A Report from the National Asthma Education and Prevention Program Coordinating Committee Expert Panel Working Group. J Allergy Clin Immunol. 2020;146(6):1217.*)

prescribed, and goals of therapy. A written asthma action plan is a useful resource and may be required at school.

Patients should be trained to use their inhalers correctly, and this training should be reviewed at future visits. Twice daily home monitoring with a peak flow meter is helpful for patients with severe asthma to identify early signs of exacerbation. Identification of triggers such as specific activities or allergens can help facilitate the reduction in exposure to known triggers. Patients should not be exposed to cigarette smoke or vaping. Vaccination against respiratory pathogens may prevent severe exacerbations.[14]

SUMMARY

Asthma is a common, chronic disease that can present in childhood. Recognition of risk factors and signs are important for early detection, diagnosis, and treatment. Treatment is guided by stepwise use of medications that target both symptoms and prevention. Patients and their parents play key roles in monitoring symptoms and preventing worsening asthma. An asthma specialist can facilitate advanced therapies for patients with more severe symptoms.

CLINICS CARE POINTS

- When a patient has had multiple episodes of wheezing, rule out asthma.
- Wheezing does not always mean asthma, and asthma does not always cause wheezing.
- It is easier to gain control of a small fire than a raging forest fire. Treat asthma early to prevent it from escalating out of control.
- In an allergic asthma patient, exposure to allergens can be like sparks on a pile of dry wood. Try to reduce exposure to things that could light the fire!
- Using daily preventative medications is like lightly misting the dry logs with water. Infrequent application still allows sparks to light the wood, but gradually soaked wood has a harder time being lit by sparks.
- If a patient or parent is concerned about regular use of inhaled steroids, it is important to educate about relative doses of inhaled (topical) steroids vs oral steroids.

DISCLOSURE

The author has no commercial or financial conflicts of interest related to the subjects of this article. No funding sources have been allotted for the publication of this article.

REFERENCES

1. Sherenian MG, Biagini Myers JM, Martin LJ, et al. The pediatric asthma risk score (PARS): making the move to the most accurate pediatric asthma risk screening tool. Expert Rev Clin Immunol 2019;15(11):1115–8.
2. Inserro A. CDC Study Puts Economic Burden of Asthma at More Than $80 Billion Per Year. 2018. Available at: https://www.ajmc.com/view/cdc-study-puts-economic-burden-of-asthma-at-more-than-80-billion-per-year. Accessed November 13, 2022.
3. Nurmagambetov T, Kuwahara R, Garbe, P. The Economic Burden of Asthma in the United States, 2008 - 2013. 2017. Available at: https://www.thoracic.org/about/newsroom/press-releases/resources/asthma-costs-in-us.pdf. Accessed November 13, 2022.

4. Naja AS, Permaul P, Phipatanakul W. Taming asthma in school-aged children: a comprehensive review. J Allergy Clin Immunol Pract 2018;6(3):726–35.

5. Childhood Asthma (Pediatric Asthma) Defined. Available at: https://www.aaaai.org/Tools-for-the-Public/Allergy,-Asthma-Immunology-Glossary/Childhood-Asthma-(Pediatric-Asthma)-Defined. Accessed November 20, 2022.

6. Chang TS, Lemanske RF Jr, Guilbert TW, et al. Evaluation of the modified asthma predictive index in high-risk preschool children. J Allergy Clin Immunol Pract 2013;1(2):152–6.

7. Biagini Meyers JM, Schauberger E, He H, et al. A pediatric asthma risk score to better predict asthma development in young children. J Allergy Clin Immunol 2019;143(5):1803–10.

8. Pediatric Asthma Risk Score. Available at: https://pars.research.cchmc.org/. Accessed November 30, 2022.

9. Asthma Overview. Available at: https://www.aaaai.org/Conditions-Treatments/Asthma/Asthma-Overview. Accessed November 20, 2022.

10. Mild, Moderate, Severe Asthma: What Do Grades Mean?. Available at: https://www.healthychildren.org/English/health-issues/conditions/allergies-asthma/Pages/Mild-Moderate-Severe-Asthma-What-Do-Grades-Mean.aspx#:~:text=In%20making%20a%20decision%20about,%2C%20moderate%2C%20or%20severe%20asthma.

11. Sawicki G, Haver K. Asthma in children younger than 12 years: Overview of initiating therapy and monitoring control. UpToDate. Available at: https://www.uptodate.com/contents/asthma-in-children-younger-than-12-years-overview-of-initiating-therapy-and-monitoring-control/print?search=Irr&topicRef=99489&source=see_link. Accessed November 10, 2022.

12. Lui AH, Zeiger RS, Sorkness CA, et al. The Childhood Asthma Control Test*: Retrospective determination and clinical validation of a cut point to identify children with very poorly controlled asthma, J Allergy Clin Immunol, 126 (2), 2010, 267-273. Available at: https://www.jacionline.org/article/S0091-6749(10)00887-0/fulltext. Accessed July 26, 2023.

13. 2020 Focused updates to the asthma management guidelines: a report from the national asthma education and prevention program coordinating committee expert panel working group. J Allergy Clin Immunol 2020;146(6):1217.

14. 2022 GINA Main Report. Available at: https://ginasthma.org/gina-reports/. Accessed January 22, 2023.

15. Choi J, Azmat CE. Leukotriene Receptor Antagonists. (Updated 2022 Dec 3). In: StatPearls (Internet). Treasure Island (FL): StatPearls Publishing; 2022 Jan-. Available at: https://www.ncbi.nlm.nih.gov/books/NBK554445/. Accessed January 22, 2023.

Update on Allergy Diagnostics

Tara Bruner, MHS, PA-C, DFAAPA[a],*, Scott Duhaime, MPAS, PA-C[b]

KEYWORDS

- Blood allergy • In vitro allergy • Specific IgE testing
- Component-resolved diagnostics • Food allergy • Pet allergy

KEY POINTS

- In vitro blood allergy testing helps clinicians evaluate patients with allergies, whether it be respiratory allergies or food allergies all within the context of patient symptoms.
- Diagnosing patients with food allergies can be aided using component-resolved diagnostics by evaluating cross-reactivity of proteins, proteins, stability, and pan allergens.
- Allergy component-resolved diagnostics are available for food allergy, pet allergy, Hymenoptera allergy, and alpha-Gal.

UPDATE IN ALLERGY DIAGNOSTICS

A diagnosis of an immunoglobulin E (IgE)-mediated allergy is made based on a detailed clinical history, physical findings, and testing, for example, specific IgE sensitization test (in vitro blood test or skin prick tests) and at times an oral food challenge.[1] The testing for IgE sensitization has traditionally been based on extracts of the allergen sources but in the last decade, using molecular allergology through component-resolved diagnostics (CRD) has become more common in clinical practice. The definition of CRD is the in vitro detection of specific IgE to individual molecules of the whole allergen either recombinant or purified native allergens.[2] The more traditional routes of allergy detection have been through skin prick test, which started back in the 1800s and has evolved over time. With a discovery of IgE in 1967 blood allergy testing has improved during the decades with improvement into a solid phase in vitro detection to automated and, now, for the past 2 decades into CRD.[3] This trend will continue as more and more allergy components are introduced to the United States from other parts of the world, particularly Europe, where molecular allergology is considered a cornerstone of diagnosing allergic disease.[4]

[a] ImmunoDiagnostics, Thermo Fisher Scientific, 164 Lamar Lane, Searcy, AR 72143, USA; [b] Otolaryngology-Allergy, Thermo Fisher Scientific, 519 Roble Vista, San Antonio, TX 78258, USA
* Corresponding author. 4169 Commercial Avenue, Portage, MI 49002.
E-mail address: Tara.bruner@thermofisher.com

Physician Assist Clin 8 (2023) 663–673
https://doi.org/10.1016/j.cpha.2023.05.002
2405-7991/23/Published by Elsevier Inc.

physicianassistant.theclinics.com

Traditional extract-based IgE blood tests measure the whole extract (all the components) of a particular allergen source, where molecular allergology measures the individual components (or proteins) of the allergen. Some of these individual components within a whole allergen are more likely to lead to a systemic allergic response, some are more indicative of cross-reactivity and may only cause a mild, nonsystemic response, susceptibility to denaturing, or no reaction at all.[4] Understanding the relationship between the patient history, physical examination, whole allergen (blood test or skin prick test), and the available individual components can assist the clinician in making a more accurate diagnosis and guiding medical management and treatment.[4] The in vitro assay of molecular allergy or component-resolved diagnostic testing aids in the understanding of cross-reactivity, patient risk and patient management and immunotherapy.[4]

Current commercially available components used in the clinic (in the United States) to aid in the diagnosis of food allergy include, peanut, tree-nuts (hazelnut, walnut, Brazil nut, cashew), wheat, and sesame. There are also components available, not to aid in the diagnosis but to aid in the treatment planning for tolerating baked milk and egg. In addition to food components, there are also CRD available for cat, dog, and horse, which can reveal true primary sensitizations as opposed to cross-reactivity between species, and even distinguishing primary sensitization between male and female dogs. Other components include stinging insects, distinguishing between honeybee, yellow jacket, and paper wasp. Finally, there is the single component of alpha-Gal, which is used to aid in the diagnosis of alpha-gal syndrome[5] (**Fig. 1**).

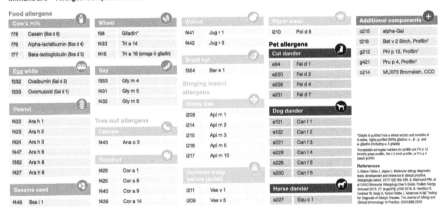

Fig. 1. Components available and Food and Drug Administration approved within the United States for common allergic triggers.

Allergen and allergen components nomenclature is governed by the World Health Organization and the International Union of Immunological Sciences.[6] The name of each allergen component is based on the Latin name of the allergen source (the first 3 letters of the first word and the first letter of the second). The allergen component is also given a number based on the order of discovery.[6]

For example, one of the peanut components is Ara h 2, which is derived from *Arachis hypogaea*, and is the second to be discovered but not necessarily the second in any scale of likelihood of causing reaction. The laboratory results may also include the letters "n" or "r," which indicate the source of the allergen component whether native or recombinant.[7]

CRD differ based on the proteins and protein families. For milk and egg components, the proteins are either stable or denaturable with extensive heating. Peanut and tree nut components relate with the individual protein families and cross-reactivity.

MILK

The components significant for cow's milk that drive clinical reactivity are characterized by protein stability. There are 3 approved CRD proteins within cow's milk that impact clinical reactivity. The protein casein is a stable protein due to its structure and unique protein sequence. It is unlikely to denature with extensive heating and or gastric acid; therefore, the baking process will not change the diagnosis of milk allergy.[8] There are 2 other proteins α-lactalbumin and β-lactoglobulin that are labile proteins for milk. These proteins can be denatured with extensive heating, which is defined at 350° for 30 minutes.[9] Any of these 3 proteins will cause the whole allergen (skin prick or whole allergen IgE) to be positive. If a patient has positivity to the labile proteins (α-lactalbumin and β-lactoglobulin) and negative to the stable protein (casein), a food challenge could reveal the patient is tolerant to the baked product. Similarly, if a patient is positive for casein but negative or positive for the labile proteins, it would be expected that such a patient would fail a food challenge to the baked milk (**Fig. 2**).[9] Identification of these components, determine whether a patient can potentially tolerate baked milk foods or avoid all forms of food containing milk.[9] Allergen testing with CRD along with whole allergen milk allows for informed decision-making and consideration for referral to an allergist for a possible oral food challenge and or potential lifelong avoidance.

EGG COMPONENTS

There are 2 components available for the management of patients with hen's egg allergy. The stable protein is ovomucoid, and the labile protein is ovalbumin, which is

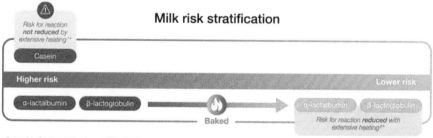

Fig. 2. Milk components.

denaturable.[10] Protein denaturing is a possibility for the ovalbumin when extensively heated, which could potentially allow a patient to tolerate baked forms of egg in the absence of the stable protein (ovomucoid) (**Fig. 3**). There is a potential for a patient to become tolerant of eggs in all forms as time progresses and egg is safely introduced in the diet.[10]

The different components in whole allergens of different species may sound daunting at first but fortunately the components themselves are usually grouped into individual protein families that display similar characteristics.

PEANUT AND TREE NUT COMPONENTS

When speaking of peanut and tree nut components, it is important to know the protein family it originates from. Such as seed storage proteins, these can be associated with systemic response (**Fig. 4**).

STORAGE PROTEINS

There is a spectrum these proteins fall into, with cross-reactivity at one end with limited risk for systemic response and the seed storage proteins that carry a risk of systemic response at the other end (**Fig. 5**). Along that spectrum are additional families of proteins that can be cross-reactive with other proteins in nature or be associated with a localized reaction, or oral pollen syndrome (food pollen syndrome).[11,12]

PEANUT

The current available peanut CRD include Ara h 1, Ara h 2, Ara h 3, Ara h 6, Ara h 8, and Ara h 9. Peanut (and tree nut) components are defined as primary sensitization and cross-reactivity between proteins.[11–13] Those components present in foods and other plant-based foods and pollen allergens are cross-reactive proteins.[14] In addition, tree nut CRD are available for hazelnut, walnut, Brazil nut, and cashew nut.

The discussion centers on the proteins within the whole allergen that drive clinical reactivity with a risk of systemic, localized, or no clinical response.[15,16]

The seed storage proteins for peanuts are Ara h 1, Ara h 2, Ara h 3, and Ara h 6. These proteins are unique in structure and are stable to heat and digestion.[17] These proteins indicate primary sensitization to peanuts along the risk ramp. Stepping down the risk ramp are the lipid transfer proteins (LTPs). Ara h 9 is a component stable to heat and digestion, associated with local and systemic reactions and can have some cross-reactivity with stone fruits.[12,16] Risk of systemic reaction decreases and protein cross reactivity increases as progression to the the PR-10 protein family.

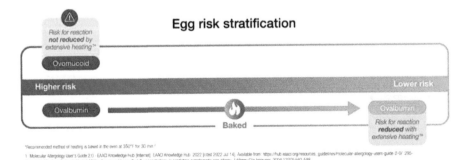

Fig. 3. Egg components.

Characteristics of allergen families[1]

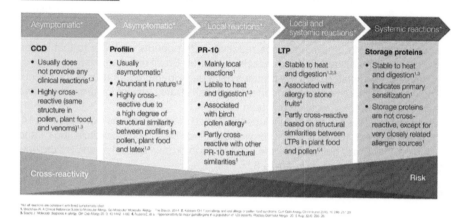

Fig. 4. Characteristics of allergen families.

For peanut this is the Ara h 8 protein. This plant protein is labile to heat and digestion and often cause localized reaction associated with oral allergy syndrome (food pollen syndrome).[6,15] These can also be predictive on not having clinical reactivity.[15]

The protein sequence of Ara h 8 is very similar to that found in birch pollen Bet V 2.[13] A birch pollen-sensitized patient can exhibit a positive whole allergen peanut diagnostic test, and if absent to the sensitization of the storage proteins, the patient may pass and tolerate a peanut food challenge.[15]

The left of **Fig. 5** shows the risk of systemic reaction is low while the level of cross-reactivity increases. These protein families are ubiquitous in nature also called pan allergens. Both profilin and cross-reactive carbohydrate determinants (CCD) are prevalent in nature and can be present in whole peanut extract, and much like the birch

Assessing risk[1-3]

Peanut and tree nut components	CCD	Profilin*	PR-10	LTP	Storage proteins
Peanut	MUXF3	Bet v 2	Ara h 8	Ara h 9	Ara h 1, 2, 3, 6
Hazelnut	MUXF3	Bet v 2	Cor a 1	Cor a 8	Cor a 9,14
Walnut	MUXF3	Bet v 2		Jug r 3	Jug r 1
Brazil nut	MUXF3	Bet v 2			Ber e 1
Cashew	MUXF3	Bet v 2			Ana o 3

Cross-reactivity / Risk

Fig. 5. Peanut and Tree Nut Components risk ramp.

pollen-sensitized patient, if also absent to sensitization of the storage proteins, these patients may successfully pass an oral food challenge to peanuts.[14,18]

TREE NUT COMPONENTS

The conversation of component cross-reactivity with peanuts is similar to that in tree nuts. The components available for hazelnut, walnut, Brazil nut, and cashew nut proteins have been identified, and the proteins have been identified. Similar to the peanut example on the risk ramp, the components can risk stratify, risk of systemic response versus potential cross-reactivity bewteen proteins.

The available CRDs for hazelnut include the 2 seed storage proteins Cor a 9, Cor a 14, LTP Cor a 8, and PR-10 Cor a 1.[19,20] For walnut include seed storage protein Jug r 1 and LTP Jug r 3.[16,21] Brazil nut includes the seed storage protein Ber e 1,[22] and for cashew nut, the seed storage protein is Ana o 3.[23]

SESAME COMPONENTS

The available CRDs for sesame seed includes the seed storage protein Ses i 1. This component enhances the diagnosis of sesame allergy due to higher sensitivity and specificity than whole sesame testing.[24]

WHEAT COMPONENTS

Component-resolved diagnostic testing available for wheat is Tri a 19 (Gliadin) storage protein Tri a 14 LTP and n-Gliadin. Wheat allergy can be composed of different clinical manifestations ranging from wheat hypersensitivity (IgE food allergy such as anaphylaxis, baker's asthma, contact urticaria, and wheat-dependent exercise-induced anaphylaxis, WDEIA) to autoimmune conditions (celiac) and nonautoimmune/nonallergic (gluten sensitivity).[25,26] Components of the wheat whole allergen IgE can help us sort out some of the wheat hypersensitivity and improve the accuracy of the diagnosis.

There are some components of the wheat whole allergen IgE that are not consistently well represented in the whole allergen test (whole allergen-specific IgE or skin prick test extract). Testing the whole allergen and wheat components together not only increases the specificity of the testing but also adds to the sensitivity because the additional components will complete the patient's wheat allergen sensitization profile.[26]

In addition to the whole allergen, which should reflex when positive to the components just described, an additional order of gliadin components will add to the overall sensitivity of the testing by testing for the 4 gliadin components not represented well in the whole extract: alpha, beta, gamma, and omega 5 gliadin (Tri a 19). Any of which could be responsible for the WDEIA but most ascribed to the omega 5 gliadin.[26]

Food allergy components resolved diagnostic testing aids in the understanding of cross-reactivity, patient risk and patient management, and immunotherapy.[4] See **Table 1** for food allergen, allergen component, component family, and interpretation considerations.

PET COMPONENTS

Pet CRD provides a more precise diagnosis and understanding of the primary animal sensitizer. The clinical value is how pet components predict asthma severity, asthma phenotyping, and assist with patient management and pet selection. There is a variety of protein families involved in pet resolved components.

Table 1
Food allergen components

Food Allergen	Allergen Component	Component Family	Interpretation
Cow's milk	Bos d 8	Casein	Heat stable, risk of severe reaction, Avoid cow's milk
	Bos d 4	Alpha-lactalbumin	Heat liable, consider baked food, challenge
	Bos d 5	Beta-lactoglobulin	Heat liable, consider baked food, challenge
Hen's egg	Gal d 1	Ovomucoid	Heat stable, risk of severe reaction, Avoid Hen's egg
	Gal d 2	Ovalbumin	Heat liable, consider baked food, challenge
Peanut	Ara h 1, 2, 3, 6	Storage protein	Risk of severe reaction, avoid peanuts
	Ara h 8	PR-10 protein	Cross-reactive with birch pollen, consider food challenge
	Ara h 9	LTP	Cross-reactive with stone fruits, consider food challenge
Hazelnut	Cor a 9, 14	Storage protein	Risk of severe reaction, avoid hazelnut
	Cor a 1	PR-10 protein	Cross-reactive, consider oral food challenge
	Cor a 8	LTP	Cross-reactive, consider oral food challenge
Walnut	Jug r 1	Storage protein	Risk of severe reaction, avoid walnuts
	Jug r 3	LTP	Cross-reactive, consider oral food challenge
Brazil nut	Ber e 1	Storage protein	Risk of severe reaction, avoid brazil nut
Cashew nut	Ana o 3	Storage protein	Risk of severe reaction, avoid cashew nut
Wheat	Tri a 14	LTP	Cross-reactive, consider oral food challenge
	Tri a 19	Storage protein	Risk of severe reaction, avoid wheat
	N-gliadin	Storage protein	Risk of severe reaction, avoid wheat
Sesame seed	Ses i 1	Storage protein	Risk of severe reaction, avoid sesame

Within the whole allergen of cat dander, there is Fel d 1. Fel d 1 is species specific to cat and is the majority of proteins found in cat dander.[27] It is a unique cat-specific marker of sensitization and a secretoglobin and the major cat allergen expressed in the skin and salivary glands.[27]

Other proteins are associated with cat as listed in **Fig. 6**. The colored bar through the protein represents the potential for cross-reactivity within that family of proteins. Fel d 2 is a serum albumin and cross-reactive with that of dog Can f 3.[4] Serum albumins are highly cross-reactive molecules and considered abundant minor antigens yet are known to be less concerning for driving clinical respiratory symptoms.[4] Additionally, Fel d 4 and Fel d 7 are lipocalin proteins and are the most important allergen protein family and major allergens synthesized by the salivary glands and dispersed in the environment via saliva and dander. These proteins can also be cross-reactive with other

Species-specific or cross-reactive?[1,2]

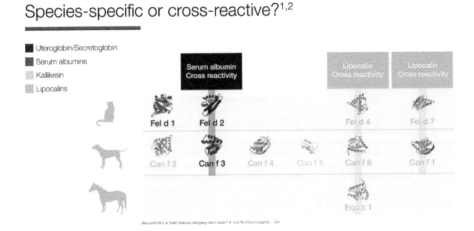

Fig. 6. Pet CRD.

lipocalin proteins found in dog and even horse, see **Fig. 6**. These proteins can drive clinical reactivity but also have the potential for cross-reactivity with other lipocalins.[4]

There are also dog component proteins unique to the canine species, 2 lipocalin components, Can f 2 and Can f 4.[4] There is a unique component for dogs, Can f 5. It is a prostatic Kallikrein that is isolated from the urine of male dogs and considered a major allergen.[4] Patient sensitized only to Can f 5 may tolerate female dogs.[4] Can f 5 also can manifest as a clinically relevant cross-reactive allergy with human seminal fluid.[28]

Cross-reactivity found within the proteins between species can help determine which animal is responsible for driving patient symptoms. It also clarifies which immunotherapy or management tool is best for the patient.[29] Additionally, the value of understanding pet components is its ability to help predict asthma severity and development.[28] Greater than 3 positive pet components correlate with increasing asthma severity.[30]

HYMENOPTERA COMPONENTS

Hymenoptera allergen components are available for honeybee, common wasp (yellow jacket), and paper wasp. Component-resolved IgE tests use recombinant venom allergens that may improve specificity to determine genuine species or double sensitization to both honeybee and wasp allergy.[31] The Hymenoptera recombinant components remove the pan allergen CCD, reducing cross-reactivity[4] (**Fig. 7**).

The detection of specific IgE to wasp and honeybee component proteins helps determine genuine double sensitization and cross-reactivity. Moreover, there are components in honeybee that are underrepresented in the whole extract; however, through CRD, they are detectable and predict patients' success with immunotherapy.[32]

ALPHA-GAL COMPONENT

There is a food allergy to red meat that is driven by alpha-Gal. This delayed reaction may occur hours after ingestion of mammalian red meat. Patients have IgE antibodies to the carbohydrate alpha-Gal that seems to be acquired via tick bites. CRD to alpha-Gal in the blood is the preferred method of diagnosis. The IgE antibodies to galactose-α-1,3-galactose is an oligosaccharide present in mammals except humans and old

Component testing allows more precise diagnostics

i1 Honey Bee   i3 Common Wasp (Yellow Jacket)   i4 Paper Wasp

Api m 1	Phospholipase A2
Api m 2	Hyaluronidase
Api m 3	Acid Phosphatase
Api m 5	Dipeptidyl Peptidase
Api m 10	Icarapin

| Ves v 1 | Phospholipase A1 |
| Ves v 5 | Antigen 5 |

| Pol d 5 | Antigen 5 |

Adapted from S. Blank, M. B. Bilo, M. Ollert Component-resolved diagnostics to direct in venom immunotherapy: Important steps towards precision medicine Clin Exp Allergy 2018;48.p357 2018

Fig. 7. Hymenoptera components.

world monkeys.[33] Increase in serum IgE to alpha-Gal following a tick bite from the Ixodidae family of hard ticks specifically in the United States the Lone Star tick *Amblyomma americanum* are the predominant carriers causing alpha-Gal sensitization.[34] This can present as an allergy to mammalian meat specifically beef, pork, and lamb and game but not to chicken, turkey, or fish.[35] The value of component testing for alpha-Gal can include specific IgE testing to those mammalian meats as well for confirmatory diagnosis.

SUMMARY

Precise molecular diagnostics for allergy allow more in-depth analysis of sensitization to allergens providing anaphylactic risk assessment, personalized management and immunotherapy choices, and overall patient care. "Component resolved diagnostics allows a detailed molecular profile in a polyclonal IgE repertoire of the allergic patient."[4] The need for allergy medicine has been on the increase worldwide. Fortunately, the burden of the increased demand has been met not only with the allergist but also the primary care providers and otolaryngologist, thus creating a team of medical providers united to meet the challenge. The use of whole allergen diagnostics, skin prick testing and serum-specific IgE testing, allows for some but not all the diagnostic and laboratory strength needed in this quest to meet the demand. CRD testing, which adds to the armamentarium of the legacy diagnostics, provides the allergy team to decode the complex allergy patients facing the medical community. All of this relies on the allergy team understanding the knowledge and utility of components from the science to the clinical application and best practices. As more and more components are developed and cleared for use in the United States, there will be an ongoing need for education and training in their use.

CLINICS CARE POINTS

- Component Allergy Testing is a simple blood test to aid in the diagnosis of allergic diseases when clinical symptoms are present.
- Component resolved allergy testing helps risk stratify patients for allergic diseases.

DISCLOSURE

T. Bruner and S. Duhaime are employees of Thermo Fisher Scientific manufacturer of the ImmunoCAP-specific IgE diagnostic blood test.

REFERENCES

1. Bird JA. Approach to evaluation and management of a patient with multiple food allergies. Allergy Asthma Proc 2016;37(2):86–91.
2. Calamelli E, Liotti L, Beghetti I, et al. Component-resolved diagnosis in food allergies. Medicina (Lithuania) 2019;55(8):498.
3. Platts-Mills TAE, Heymann PW, Commins SP, et al. The discovery of IgE 50 years later. Ann Allergy Asthma Immunol 2016;116(3):179–82.
4. Matricardi PM, Kleine-Tebbe J, Hoffmann HJ, et al. EAACI Molecular Allergology User's Guide. Pediatr Allergy Immunol 2016;27:1–250.
5. Thermo Fisher Scientific Allergy and Autoimmune Disease. ImmunoCAP Allergen Components. Available at: https://www.thermofisher.com/phadia/us/en/our-solutions/immunocap-allergy-solutions/specific-ige-single-allergens/allergen-components.html. Accessed November 27, 2022.
6. Canonica GW, Ansotegui IJ, Pawankar R, et al. A WAO-ARIA-GA2LEN consensus document on molecular-based allergy diagnostics. World Allergy Organ J 2013;6(1).
7. Hoffmann-Sommergruber K. Proteomics and its impact on food allergy diagnosis. EuPA Open Proteom 2016;12:10–2.
8. Shek LPC, Bardina L, Castro R, et al. Humoral and cellular responses to cow milk proteins in patients with milk-induced IgE-mediated and non-IgE-mediated disorders. Allergy 2005;60(7):912–9.
9. Nowak-Wegrzyn A, Bloom KA, Sicherer SH, et al. Tolerance to extensively heated milk in children with cow's milk allergy. J Allergy Clin Immunol 2008;122(2):342–7.
10. Benhamou AH, Caubet JC, Eigenmann PA, et al. State of the art and new horizons in the diagnosis and management of egg allergy. Allergy 2010;65(3):283–9.
11. Asarnoj A, Nilsson C, Lidholm J, et al. Peanut component Ara h 8 sensitization and tolerance to peanut. J Allergy Clin Immunol 2012;130(2):468–72.
12. Lauer I, Dueringer N, Pokoj S, et al. The non-specific lipid transfer protein, Ara h 9, is an important allergen in peanut. Clin Exp Allergy 2009;39(9):1427–37.
13. Mittag D, Akkerdaas J, Ballmer-Weber BK, et al. Ara h 8, a Bet v 1-homologous allergen from peanut, is a major allergen in patients with combined birch pollen and peanut allergy. J Allergy Clin Immunol 2004;114(6):1410–7.
14. Katelaris CH. Food allergy and oral allergy or pollen-food syndrome. Curr Opin Allergy Clin Immunol 2010;10(3):246–51.
15. Nucera E, Mezzacappa S, Aruanno A, et al. Original paper Hypersensitivity to major panallergens in a population of 120 patients. Adv Dermatol Allergol 2015;4:255–61.
16. Sastre J. Molecular diagnosis in allergy. Clin Exp Allergy 2010;40(10):1442–60.
17. Peeters KABM, Koppelman SJ, van Hoffen E, et al. Does skin prick test reactivity to purified allergens correlate with clinical severity of peanut allergy? Clin Exp Allergy 2007;37(1):108–15.
18. Bradshaw N. Go Molecular! A Clinical Reference Guide to Molecular Allergy; 2021. Available at: https://www.thermofisher.com/diagnostic-education/dam/commercial/library-resources/UK%20Go%20Molecular%20%20The%20Basics%20(Part%201)%20-%202021.pdf. Accessed June 26, 2023.

19. Kattan JD, Sicherer SH, Sampson HA. Clinical reactivity to hazelnut may be better identified by component testing than traditional testing methods. J Allergy Clin Immunol Pract 2014;2(5):633–4.e1.

20. Masthoff LJN, Mattsson L, Zuidmeer-Jongejan L, et al. Sensitization to Cor a 9 and Cor a 14 is highly specific for a hazelnut allergy with objective symptoms in Dutch children and adults. J Allergy Clin Immunol 2013;132(2):393–9.

21. Roux KH, Teuber SS, Sathe SK. Tree nut allergens. Int Arch Allergy Immunol 2003;131(4):234–44.

22. Pastorello EA, Farioli L, Pravettoni V, et al. Sensitization to the major allergen of Brazil nut is correlated with the clinical expression of allergy. J Allergy Clin Immunol 1998;102(6 Pt 1):1021–7.

23. Uotila R, Kukkonen AK, Blom WM, et al. Component-resolved diagnostics demonstrates that most peanut-allergic individuals could potentially introduce tree nuts to their diet. Clin Exp Allergy 2018;48(6):712–21.

24. Maruyama N, Nakagawa T, Ito K, et al. Measurement of specific IgE antibodies to Ses i 1 improves the diagnosis of sesame allergy. Clin Exp Allergy 2016;46(1): 163–71.

25. Hofmann SC, Fischer J, Eriksson C, et al. IgE detection to $\alpha/\beta/\gamma$-gliadin and its clinical relevance in wheat-dependent exercise-induced anaphylaxis. Allergy 2012;67(11):1457–60.

26. Palacin A, Varela J, Quirce S, et al. Recombinant lipid transfer protein Tri a 14: A novel heat and proteolytic resistant tool for the diagnosis of baker's asthma. Clin Exp Allergy 2009;39(8):1267–76.

27. Bonnet B, Messaoudi K, Jacomet F, et al. An update on molecular cat allergens: Fel d 1 and what else? Chapter 1: Fel d 1, the major cat allergen. Allergy Asthma Clin Immunol 2018;14(1).

28. Dávila I, Domínguez-Ortega J, Navarro-Pulido A, et al. Consensus document on dog and cat allergy. Allergy 2018;73(6):1206–22.

29. Konradsen JR, Fujisawa T, van Hage M, et al. Allergy to furry animals: New insights, diagnostic approaches, and challenges. J Allergy Clin Immunol 2015; 135(3):616–25.

30. Patelis A, Gunnbjornsdottir M, Alving K, et al. Allergen extract vs. component sensitization and airway inflammation, responsiveness and new-onset respiratory disease. Clin Exp Allergy 2016;46(5):730–40.

31. Spillner E, Blank S, Jakob T. Hymenoptera allergens: From venom to "venome". Front Immunol 2014;5:77.

32. Köhler J, Blank S, Müller S, et al. Component resolution reveals additional major allergens in patients with honeybee venom allergy. J Allergy Clin Immunol 2014; 133(5):1383–9.

33. Commins SP, James HR, Kelly LA, et al. The relevance of tick bites to the production of IgE antibodies to the mammalian oligosaccharide galactose-α-1,3-galactose. J Allergy Clin Immunol 2011;127(5):1286–93.e6.

34. Macher BA, Galili U. The Galα1,3Galβ1,4GlcNAc-R (α-Gal) Epitope: A Carbohydrate of Unique Evolution and Clinical Relevance.; 2008.

35. Commins SP, Satinover SM, Hosen J, et al. Delayed anaphylaxis, angioedema, or urticaria after consumption of red meat in patients with IgE antibodies specific for galactose-α-1,3-galactose. J Allergy Clin Immunol 2009;123(2):426–33.

Food Allergy, Oral Food Challenges, and Oral Immunotherapy

Tina L.R. Dominguez, PA-C, MMS[a,b,c,]*

KEYWORDS

- Oral food challenge • Food allergy • Food allergens • Allergy testing
- Skin prick testing • Food-specific IgE testing • Component testing

KEY POINTS

- A double-blind placebo-controlled food challenge is the gold standard for diagnosis of food allergy, but open food challenges are most commonly done in clinical practice.
- Oral food challenges can be rewarding and a valuable educational experience, regardless of outcome.
- When deciding to conduct an oral food challenge, there are various patient factors to consider.
- Skin prick testing, serum immunoglobulin E testing, and component testing can all be used to help clinicians predict outcomes of oral food challenges.

INTRODUCTION

The prevalence of food allergies has quickly become an epidemic and global health concern for many families in the last decade. As a potentially life-threatening disease, food allergies have thus become one of the main topics of conversation in allergy and asthma. Affecting over 32 million people in the United States alone, it is a burden not only to the families but also to the health care system as a whole.

One in 13 children suffers from a food allergy, and about 40% are allergic to more than one food allergen.[1] More than one-half of adults with food allergies have experienced an anaphylactic reaction.[1] Many of them suffer a diminished quality of life and oftentimes believe hopeless and isolated. Although food allergy research has made great strides in the last decade, there is still a lack of knowledge surrounding the full impact of food allergies, including the true cost to our health care system. From 2007 and 2016, insurance claims for food allergy anaphylaxis have increased 377% and are undoubtedly higher today.[2] The current estimated yearly cost of $25 billion

[a] Latitude Food Allergy Care, 2303 Camino Ramon Suite 150, San Ramon, CA 94583, USA;
[b] Aimmune Therapeutics; [c] Sean N. Parker Center for Allergy & Asthma Research
* 525 Olympic Avenue, Hayward, CA 94544.
E-mail addresses: tdominguez.pa@gmail.com; tdominguez@latitudefac.com

Physician Assist Clin 8 (2023) 675–684
https://doi.org/10.1016/j.cpha.2023.05.003
2405-7991/23/© 2023 Elsevier Inc. All rights reserved.

physicianassistant.theclinics.com

includes the direct cost to the health care system and the costs that food allergy families are burdened with; however, the exact cost of food allergies is difficult to measure.[2]

DIAGNOSIS

A food allergy is the result of abnormal immune response to a food that causes an adverse reaction. Serum (immunoglobulin [Ig]E) testing and skin prick testing are widely used to diagnose food allergies, but testing alone does not confirm the diagnosis. The patient's clinical history, serum IgE, and skin prick testing can assist in making the diagnosis; however, an oral food challenge (OFC) is the criterion standard for diagnosing food allergies. Keep in mind that when evaluating a patient for food allergies, it is important to focus testing on the specific foods that triggered a reaction and avoid multi-food testing. Testing for foods that a patient is already able to consume without reaction can lead to unnecessary avoidance of a food they have been tolerating due to false-positive test results.

Of the various types of OFCs, there is one that is truly considered the gold standard test; however, due to its complexity, the double-blind placebo-controlled food challenge (DBPCFC) is generally only performed in clinic research trials. A DBPCFC requires the patient and the challenge administrator to be blinded. Each food must be challenged on separate days with an additional day for the placebo; however, these challenges are cumbersome and require a lot of time and preparation and are not practical in a nonresearch setting.

Single-blind placebo food challenges are similar to the double-blind placebo food challenge with only the patient blinded and in most cases do not include a placebo challenge but are still difficult to perform in a nonresearch setting. The most convenient and regularly performed challenge in clinical practice is an open OFC. In an open OFC, both the provider and patient are unblinded, thus only requiring that each food allergen be challenged on separate days, without a placebo day.

According to prior studies, the OFC is widely underused. The American Academy of Allergy, Asthma and Immunology Adverse Reactions to Food Committee surveyed a total of 546 allergy providers in 2020.[3] Based on the findings of the survey, there were significantly more providers offering OFCs compared with respondents in 2009, 95% compared with the previous 84.5%.[3] Many practices perform more than 10 OFCs per month, 17% compared with 5.6% in 2009.[3]

OFCs have been shown to improve the quality of life in patients and their caregivers regardless of the outcome,[4] yet somehow most practices are often still limiting the number of OFCs they are conducting due to scheduling limitations, space restrictions, staffing issues, lack of experience or proper training, the age of the patient, fear of reactions and poor outcomes, and proximity to the nearest hospital and reimbursement concerns.

CONDUCTING AN ORAL FOOD CHALLENGE
Clinical Preparedness

Patient safety is of the utmost importance when conducting an OFC and it is imperative that the clinic be prepared for any outcome.

- Conducting regular training on the management of allergic reactions and anaphylaxis ensures that everyone knows their role in the event of anaphylaxis.
- Regular inventory of emergency medications and supplies should be performed on a schedule determined by the type of supplies in the clinic and patient volume (**Table 1**).

Table 1
Emergency medications

Drug Class	Medication Name	Medication Type
Antihistamines	Cetirizine, diphenhydramine	Oral: tablet, liquid, chewable Intramuscular
H2-blockers	Famotidine	Oral: tablet, liquid, chewable
Epinephrine	1:1000 injectable multi-dose vial	Injectable
Intravenous fluids	Normal saline	—
Supplemental O$_2$	—	Oxygen tanks, pediatric and adult non-rebreather masks
Steroids	Prednisone, dexamethasone, methylprednisolone	Oral: tablet, liquid, injectable
Adrenergic bronchodilators	Albuterol	Inhaled: nebulized, hydrofluoroalkane (HFA) Inhaler
Antiemetics	Ondansetron	Oral: disintegrating

- Informing patients of the risk and benefits and obtaining consent before the start of the procedure is essential to ensure that everyone is on the same page and prepared for the visit.
- On the day of the procedure, all medication dosages should be calculated before the start of the visit to ensure that any reaction is treated in a timely and appropriate manner.[4]
- Verify the patient has their epinephrine auto-injector at the start of the visit to ensure that when the challenge is over, if a delayed reaction was to occur, they can treat the reaction accordingly.
- At the start of the visit, the clinician should verify that the patient is illness free, asthma is well controlled, perform a baseline examination, review vitals, and discuss the process with the patient and family.
- Documentation is the key for a variety of reasons, so record all dosing amounts, times, reactions, vitals, and medications given at the time of the event.

The goal of each OFC is between 4 and 5 g of protein[5]; however, for younger children, 2 to 3 g of protein is sufficient. Refer to **Table 2**, for appropriate dosing amounts based on age. In preparation of the challenge—to prevent any confusion should a reaction occur—the patient should refrain from eating or drinking anything other than water for 4 hours before the challenge.[5] Fasting can help eliminate uncertainty should a reaction occur. Although many families are careful about what they consume, accidental ingestion can occur coincidental to the appointment. For younger children, an empty stomach may also help encourage them to complete the necessary doses.[5]

A standard operating procedure can help eliminate dosing errors, take the guesswork out of trying to calculate OFC doses before the start of the visit and ensures the patient consumes the age-appropriate dose to consider the challenge a viable challenge.[1,5] Depending on the risk, a total of four or six doses are performed. Doses should be given every 15 to 30 minutes starting with 10 mg of protein. The subsequent doses are as follows, 30, 100, 300, 1000, and 3000 mg for the final dose. Higher risk challenges should increase with smaller incremental doses and longer intervals between doses.

Identifying the Appropriate Patient

When identifying the right patient and food to challenge, there are a few considerations to discuss when talking to the family about an oral challenge.[5]

Table 2
Appropriate portion sizes based on age[5]

Food Allergen	Food Used and Protein Serving Size	Age 4 mo–3 y	4–8 y	9–19+ y
Peanut/tree nuts	Peanuts/tree nuts 2g/~8 peanuts or tree nuts	—	16	16
	Peanut/tree nut butter 3g/1 tbsp	1–2 tbsp	1–2 tbsp	2 tbsp
Egg	Scrambled/hard-boiled	1/2–1 egg	1 egg	1–2 eggs
	French toast (1 egg per slice)	1/2–1 slice	1 slice	1–2 slices
Milk	Infant formula	4–8 oz	—	—
	Milk	4–8 oz	4–8 oz	8 oz
	Hard cheese	1/4–1/2 oz	1 oz	1–1 1/2 oz
	Yogurt (non-Greek style)	1/4–1/2 cup	1/2–1 cup	1/2–1 cup
Wheat	Infant cereal 1–2 g per 1/4 cup	1/4–1/2 cup	—	—
	Cooked cereal 5 g per 1/4 cup dry	1/4 cup	1/4–1/2 cup	1/4–1/2 cup
	Cooked Pasta 3g per 1/2 cup	1/4 cup	1/4–1/2 cup	1/4–1/2 cup
	Sliced bread 2–4 g per slice	1/4–1/2 slice	1/2–1 slice	1–2 slices
Fish	Cooked fish 6g/1 oz	1/2–1 oz	1 oz	2–4 oz
Shellfish	Cooked shellfish 5g/1 oz	1/2–1 oz	1 oz	2–4 oz

Data adapted from Bird et al. J Allergy clin Immunol Pract January 2020; 8(1), 75-90.

- Is home introduction of the food safe?
- Is the family afraid to introduce the food at home?
- How important is it to reintroduce or introduce the food into their diet?
  - Family is vegetarian/vegan and avoid animal products
  - Religious beliefs and avoids non-kosher foods
  - Uncommon foods: Brazil nut, macadamia
  - Other family members allergic to the food
  - Could the introduction be anxiety provoking
  - Will they be willing to keep the food in their diet?
- IgE and skin prick test not consistent with history
- Benefits of adding the food back into the diet outweigh the risks
- Assessing the tolerance of a food allergen

Patient Considerations

Shared decision-making is an integral part of OFCs. Patients should be made aware of the risks and benefits ahead of the challenge visit and consent should be obtained. There should be an open discussion about the types of reactions, how differently they are treated, how to prepare for the OFC, and what to bring to the visit. Discuss safety considerations and when an OFC may need to be postponed.[5]

- Any concurrent illness, fever, or respiratory symptoms (new onset of wheezing or cough)
- Recent use of a short acting beta-agonist within the last 48 hours

- Uncontrolled asthma, atopic dermatitis, or allergic rhinitis
- Recent allergic reaction requiring epinephrine
- Recent cardiac event and/or use of beta blockers
- Pregnancy
- Failure to discontinue the required medications listed in **Table 3**

The fear and anxiety about a reaction can be so powerful; in some cases, performing an OFC can be more harmful than beneficial and the patient's mental well-being should be taken into consideration when deciding to conduct an OFC, see **Box 1**. If they are unwilling to participate or the angst of undergoing an OFC is high, trying to conduct an OFC and determining if the outcome was due to the patient's fear and anxiety or a true allergic reaction can be quite difficult. These patients have a constant fear of the possibility of having an anaphylactic reaction and that has a crippling effect on the patients and their families. Even if the patient completes the OFC without reaction, if they are fearful of consuming the food, it is unlikely that they will continue to keep the food in their diet.

When the fear of the unknown is so high that conducting an OFC is almost impossible, the unorthodox proximity challenge may be an option to help them overcome certain fears and ultimately help them feel more comfortable with the idea of doing an OFC in time.[6,7] A proximity challenge is a way to access how a patient reacts being near the food allergen without touching or ingesting it. Research has shown that the risk of severe reaction is related to ingesting the food or contact with a mucous membrane and not through airborne, skin contact or just simply being in a room with that allergen.[6]

Shared decision-making is a key element in making any medical decision and it plays a vital role in conducting an OFC. Discussing the risks and benefits of an OFC can help guide the family in deciding if they want to pursue an OFC or not. **Table 4** outlines the potential allergic reactions that can occur during an OFC.[8]

Understanding the family's goal will help guide you and your plan. Review different case scenarios and possible outcomes. Thoroughly explain what potential reactions can occur and how each of those reactions may need to be treated. Discuss the long-term plan if they successfully complete the OFC or if a reaction occurs. Remember the value of knowing if someone is truly allergic to a food is only valuable to some and not all. Some families may opt not to do an OFC no matter how low the risk.

Determining When to Challenge: Skin Prick Testing and Food-Specific Immunoglobulin E

Determining when to challenge a food is largely based on skin prick testing, serum-specific IgE results, and clinical history; however, both tests have limitations and cannot confirm the diagnosis of a food allergy.

Table 3
Medications affecting oral food challenge outcomes[1]

Drug Class	Half-Life
Antihistamines: Oral	3–7 d
Antihistamines: Nasal	0–2 d
Antihistamines: Ophthalmic	0–2 d
H2-blockers	0–2 d
Benzodiazepines	5–7 d
Tricyclic antidepressants	2->10 d
Other	<1–14 d

> **Box 1**
> **Psychosocial aspects: is the patient and family ready?[5]**
>
> Is there a significant amount of anxiety surrounding their food allergies?
>
> Taste and/or texture aversions that would affect the challenge
>
> What is the patient's goal of the OFC?
>
> Will the patient be willing to continue to keep this food in their diet?

Skin prick testing can help predict a food allergy and is highly sensitive, but it is not specific enough to determine whether or not it is a true food allergy.[9] The benefits of skin testing are that it is relatively inexpensive compared with serum IgE testing, noninvasive, can yield immediate results and rarely produces false negatives.[9] Although most studies have shown that skin testing has a 95% predictive value, the specificity is only 74% which ultimately is not specific enough to determine how much of an allergen can be consumed before an allergic reaction or anaphylaxis would occur.[9] Skin testing alone should not be used to decide whether a food allergen should be challenged or not, but for some foods, such as buckwheat, skin prick testing is more useful than serum IgE testing in diagnosing a buckwheat allergy and when to perform an oral challenge.[10]

In addition to this, skin test results can also be affected by the type of testing supplies used and the amount of pressure applied when performing the skin test. Too little pressure and the skin test may not yield a positive, whereas too much pressure may cause a false positive in some cases. Proper training and continuous competence testing can help ensure that the test administrator can provide reliable skin prick test results. In addition to this, a patient with a history of atopic dermatitis may have falsely elevated skin prick tests as well as elevated IgE and total IgE.

Countless OFCs have been conducted for various foods and in a variety of different locations have been analyzed and have provided referenceable data points to help determine if an OFC should be done or not based on the skin prick wheal size. If the wheal exceeds the cut off, the consensus is an OFC should not be conducted or it should be conducted in a hospital setting versus in a clinical setting.[9] The data also include serum IgE cutoff values that can be used in conjunction with skin prick testing.

Serum IgE, such as skin prick testing, is another tool in the allergy providers' tool bag, and like skin prick testing, it does have its limitations and alone cannot be

Table 4
Clinical symptoms of immunoglobulin E-mediated food allergy reactions

Body System	Symptom
Skin	Flushing, pruritus, urticaria, angioedema
Eye	Pruritus, erythema, lacrimation, edema
Upper respiratory	Sneezing, rhinorrhea, congestion, hoarseness
Lower respiratory	Shortness of breath, wheezing, intercostal retractions, cough
Gastrointestinal	Nausea, vomiting, diarrhea, pain, oral angioedema, oral pruritus
Cardiovascular	Tachycardia, bradycardia, vertigo, hypotension, syncope
Nervous system	Hyperactivity, weeping, irritability, anxiety, drowsiness, loss of consciousness

used to diagnose a food allergy. Using skin prick testing and serum IgE together in addition to the history can help guide a provider in deciding if an OFC should be conducted or not.[11] **Table 5** outlines the skin prick and serum IgE cutoff values for some of the most commonly challenged foods. Although these predictive values are to be used as a guide to determine if an OFC should be conducted, history of a recent reaction or anaphylactic event outweighs the data and numerical values. Remember ingestion is the gold standard test when it comes to food allergies, if a patient has recently experienced a reaction, there is no further need to put the patient at risk for a potentially life-threatening event during an OFC.

Food Allergen Component Testing

Component testing has improved IgE testing in the last few years. Specific IgE testing for allergen components help to identify the specific protein that may cause a reaction helping to improve diagnostic accuracy by differentiating sensitization to clinically relevant versus irrelevant proteins.[13] Component testing is currently available and widely used for peanut, cashew, walnut, hazelnut, Brazil nut, egg, and milk.[13] In the case of hazelnut allergy, component testing can differentiate between true food allergies or if the elevated IgE is due to cross-reactivity with birch tree or a timothy grass allergy.[13] Unlike skin prick testing, the laboratories have to be outsourced and can take anywhere for 7 to 14 days to be resulted. For peanut, an elevated Ara h2 and Ara h 6 were associated with distinguishing a severe reaction from a mild reaction and Ana o 3 for cashew has also proven to help reduce the need for an OFC.[13]

The Oral Food Challenge

Once the decision has been made to challenge a particular food the next question is how much you should challenge. The age of the challenge participant is a key factor in determining how much protein will need to be consumed during the OFC.[5] **Table 2** can be used as a guide to help determine how much protein to challenge. This is a guide that recommends age-appropriate serving sizes for a wide variety of ages, not all patients may be able to consume the recommended dosing and others may consume much more.

Table 5 Oral food challenges positive predictive values of diagnostic testing[11,12]		
Food Allergen	**Skin Prick Wheal**	**Serum IgE**
Peanut	≥8 mm	≥15 KU/L
Tree nuts	≥8 mm	≥18 KU/L
Egg	≥10 mm	≥18 KU/L
Baked egg	≥35 mm	≥40 KU/L
Milk	≥12 mm	≥15 KU/L
Baked milk	≥35 mm	≥40 KU/L
Fish	≥20 mm	≥10 KU/L
Shellfish	≥40 mm	≥20 KU/L
Soy	≥20 mm	≥65 KU/L
Wheat	≥20 mm	≥80 KU/L
Sesame	≥8 mm	≥10 KU/L
Sunflower	≥8 mm	≥10 KU/L

Data adapted from Simberloff et al J Allergy Clin Immunol Pract March/ April 2017.

The Oral Food Challenge Outcome

Regardless of the challenge outcome, patients should have an emergency action plan and medications readily available at the time of discharge. Discuss the challenge outcome and next steps with the family. Handouts outlining these instructions or creating a template that can be added into the visit summary or patient instructions of your office visit note is invaluable to patients. Some key elements to note on the handout should include the following[5]:

- Avoid any further ingestion of the food the day of the challenge or indefinitely depending on the challenge outcome
- Limiting physical activity for the remainder of the day
- What to do should a delayed reaction occur
- Continue to carry epinephrine regardless of the challenge outcome even if there are no other food allergies
- Review proper use of epinephrine autoinjectors
- How much and how often they should be consuming that particular allergen food
- Discuss the importance of keeping the food in their diet and the risks if they do not
- Resuming any medications that were discontinued for the challenge

It is normal for a patient to feel disappointed after experiencing a reaction during a food challenge; however, it also can be a valuable learning experience in helping them recognize symptoms of an allergic reaction and experience the effectiveness of immediate treatment with epinephrine. In the end, a pass or failed OFC is a way to help answer the question of whether or not they are allergic to that particular food. It cannot tell us if they outgrew their allergy or simply were never allergic to that allergen, but ultimately, the OFC can help give these families a better understanding and can empower them with a better understanding of their food allergies.

Oral Immunotherapy

Oral Immunotherapy (OIT) helps to mitigate the risk of a moderate to severe reaction by slowly introducing the food allergen into their diet. The goal is to introduce small amounts of the food allergen with the hope that it will fly under the radar of the immune system and then slowly escalate the doses over a long period of time. Over time, OIT retrains the immune system and can decrease the risk of allergic reactions and anaphylaxis to a specific food allergen.

Research has shown that OIT can improve the quality of life for food allergy patients and their caregivers and significantly decreases stress and worry.[14,15] OIT can also reduce dietary restrictions, empowering patients to enjoy a fuller—and more satisfying—range of culinary options that helps expand their limited diet. Until recently, it was only administered in a clinical research setting; however, in 2020, arachis hypogaea (Palforzia) became the first and only Federal Drug Agency (FDA)-approved OIT for peanuts that can only be prescribed by an allergy provider.[16]

In the event of a failed OFC or if the testing indicates that a food allergen is not challengeable, OIT is something that can be offered to food allergy families. OIT is still considered an experimental treatment for some foods and should only be performed and administered in a clinical setting, under the care of an expert clinical team. Although the type of adverse reactions is similar to an OFC, there is an increased potential of a moderate to severe allergic reaction and/or anaphylaxis when compared with avoidance.[17] The increased risk of a reaction and potential risk of a life-threatening reaction should be thoroughly discussed with the patient and the family to ensure that they are aware of the risks. Although many will accept their risks to help improve their quality of life, others may not.

SUMMARY

When deciding to proceed with a food challenge, there are many factors to consider that go beyond the test values and data points. Shared decision-making is essential to any decision in health care and deciding when to challenge a food may start with you as the provider, but ultimately the decision ends with the patient and their family. As a provider, our goal is to do what is best for a patient and their family. In some families, avoidance is the answer, but for others who are data-driven the OFC is the first step in that patient's journey for answers.

DISCLOSURE

The author has nothing to disclose.

REFERENCES

1. Website: FARE - What is a Food Allergy? https://www.foodallergy.org/resources/what-food-allergy. Accessed October 20, 2022.
2. Gupta R, Holdford D, Bilaver L, et al. The economic impact of childhood food allergy in the United States. JAMA Pediatr 2013;167(11):1026–31 [published correction appears in JAMA Pediatr. 2013 Nov;167(11):1083].
3. Greiwe J, Oppenheimer J, Bird JA, et al. AAAAI Work Group Report: Trends in Oral Food Challenge Practices Among Allergists in the United States. J Allergy Clin Immunol Pract 2020;8(10):3348–55.
4. Kansen HM, Le TM, Meijer Y, et al. The impact of oral food challenges for food allergy on quality of life: A systematic review. Pediatr Allergy Immunol 2018; 29(5):527–37.
5. Bird JA, Leonard S, Groetch M, et al. Conducting an Oral Food Challenge: An Update to the 2009 Adverse Reactions to Foods Committee Work Group Report. J Allergy Clin Immunol Pract 2020;8(1):75–90.e17.
6. Dinakar C, Shroba J, Portnoy JM. The transforming power of proximity food challenges. Ann Allergy Asthma Immunol 2016;117(2):135–7.
7. Sampson HA, Gerth van Wijk R, Bindslev-Jensen C, et al. Standardizing double-blind, placebo-controlled oral food challenges: American academy of allergy, asthma & immunology-European academy of allergy and clinical immunology PRACTALL consensus report. J Allergy Clin Immunol 2012;130(6):1260–74.
8. Calvani M, Bianchi A, Reginelli C, et al. Oral Food Challenge. Medicina (Kaunas) 2019;55(10):651.
9. Sampson HA, Albergo R. Comparison of results of skin tests, RAST, and double-blind, placebo-controlled food challenges in children with atopic dermatitis. J Allergy Clin Immunol 1984;74(1):26–33.
10. Yanagida N, Sato S, Takahashi K, et al. Skin prick test is more useful than specific IgE for diagnosis of buckwheat allergy: A retrospective cross-sectional study. Allergol Int 2018;67(1):67–71.
11. Simberloff T, Parambi R, Bartnikas LM, et al. Implementation of a Standardized Clinical Assessment and Management Plan (SCAMP) for Food Challenges. J Allergy Clin Immunol Pract 2017;5(2):335–44.e3.

12. Peters RL, Gurrin LC, Allen KJ. The predictive value of skin prick testing for challenge-proven food allergy: a systematic review. Pediatr Allergy Immunol 2012;23(4):347–52.

13. Website - AAFP.org - https://www.aafp.org/dam/AAFP/documents/journals/afp/Quest_WhitePaper_ComponentTestingforFoodAllergy(v1.0).PDF. Accessed October 21, 2022.

14. Otani IM, Bégin P, Kearney C, et al. Multiple-allergen oral immunotherapy improves quality of life in caregivers of food-allergic pediatric subjects. Allergy Asthma Clin Immunol 2014;10(1):25.

15. Arasi S, Otani IM, Klingbeil E, et al. Two year effects of food allergen immunotherapy on quality of life in caregivers of children with food allergies. Allergy Asthma Clin Immunol 2014;10(1):57.

16. Patrawala S, Ramsey A, Capucilli P, et al. Real-world adoption of FDA-approved peanut oral immunotherapy with palforzia. J Allergy Clin Immunol Pract 2022; 10(4):1120–2.e1.

17. Chu DK, Wood RA, French S, et al. Oral immunotherapy for peanut allergy (PACE): a systematic review and meta-analysis of efficacy and safety. Lancet 2019;393(10187):2222–32 [published correction appears in Lancet. 2019 May 11;393(10184):1936].

Psychosocial Impacts of Allergic Disease

Amanda Michaud, DMSc, PA-C, AE-C[a],*, Tamara Hubbard, MA, LCPC[b]

KEYWORDS

- Mental health • Quality of life • Psychosocial • Asthma • Allergy • Food allergy
- Atopic dermatitis • Atopy

KEY POINTS

- There are significant psychosocial burdens for many patients and caregivers managing allergic conditions, resulting in reduced quality of life affecting emotional well-being and daily functioning.
- Atopic conditions are associated with increased risk of a variety of mental health conditions including depression, anxiety, bipolar disorder, attention-deficit hyperactivity disorder (ADHD), and emotional problems.
- Clinicians must be aware of the risk of comorbid mental health problems, screen for them, and make appropriate referrals to mental health providers when indicated.

INTRODUCTION

Allergic diseases, such as asthma, allergic rhinitis (AR), food allergy (FA), and atopic dermatitis (AD) are common conditions. Although there are known impacts on the atopic patient's physical health, there are also associations between allergic diseases and mental health.[1] Psychiatric disorders such as depression, anxiety, bipolar disorder, and attention-deficit hyperactivity disorder (ADHD) have been shown to occur more frequently in patients with allergic diseases than those without allergic diseases. Psychiatric disorders refer to clinically significant behavioral or psychosocial syndromes that cause behavioral, psychological, or biological dysfunction.[2] This article will serve to review the psychosocial burden of common allergic diseases, with focus on awareness, screening, recognition, and possible management strategies.

ALLERGIC RHINITIS

AR is a chronic inflammatory disorder that affects the nasal mucosa and causes rhinorrhea, nasal obstruction and congestion, nasal itching, and sneezing.[3] Although

[a] Family Allergy and Asthma Consultants, 4123 University Boulevard South, Suite B, Jacksonville, FL 32216, USA; [b] Tamara Hubbard, LCPC, LLC. 4160 IL Route 83, Suite 210, Long Grove, IL 60047, USA
* Corresponding author.
E-mail address: amandalmichaud@gmail.com

Physician Assist Clin 8 (2023) 685–693
https://doi.org/10.1016/j.cpha.2023.05.004
2405-7991/23/© 2023 Elsevier Inc. All rights reserved.

physicianassistant.theclinics.com

AR is a non–life-threatening condition, AR can have a major effect on quality of life (QoL).[3,4] When uncontrolled, AR has been shown to affect emotional well-being, sleep, activities of daily living, overall productivity, and school absenteeism.

Overall, patients with AR are more likely to have fatigue, mood changes, reduced cognitive functioning, depression, and anxiety.[1] Children with known atopic diseases such as AR are more likely to have emotional conduct and hyperactivity problems than those without atopic disease.[4] Children with uncontrolled AR are also more likely to have disrupted sleep, which can further exacerbate behavioral or mental health problems. In adolescents, nasal symptoms related to AR have been associated with poorer QoL.[5] Symptom severity and the presence of other atopic conditions are both associated with worse QoL.[4,5] AR has also been significantly associated with lack of concentration, increased distractibility, and lower test scores in school-age children and adolescents.[3] Adults with AR have been shown to have higher risk of psychiatric disorders such as depression and anxiety.[1]

CHRONIC RHINOSINUSITIS

Chronic rhinosinusitis (CRS) is a chronic inflammatory condition of the nose and paranasal sinuses. CRS can be associated with having nasal polyps (CRSwNP) or without nasal polyps.[6] Symptoms of CRS consist of nasal obstruction, blockage, or congestion as well as nasal discharge or drainage (anterior or posterior). Facial pain/pressure and reduced or total loss of smell can be seen. Other symptoms could include cough, headache, or fatigue.

Patients with CRS have impaired QoL, with higher risk of depression, anxiety, and sleep disruption.[7] CRS is challenging to treat and often has recurrence of disease, even after sinus surgery.[6] Many patients with CRS also have comorbid AR, which can also worsen QoL.[8] Unfortunately, many patients with CRSwNP may require surgical intervention and subsequent revision surgeries, and there is notably worse QoL in these patients, which may be reflective of more severe disease.

ASTHMA

Asthma is a respiratory condition in which the airways inflame, constrict, and produce excess mucus, making breathing difficult and triggering coughing, wheezing, and shortness of breath. The psychosocial burden of living with asthma includes limitations on daily activities, disrupted sleep, absenteeism, and increased health-care costs.[9] Poorly controlled asthma is associated with an increased risk of behavioral problems and mood disorders, such as depression and anxiety.[10,11]

The most common chronic disease of childhood, asthma affects 8.3% of children in the United States, with almost 80% of cases beginning during the first 6 years of life.[12] Asthmatic children have a significantly lower QoL than healthy children, particularly relating to physical, emotional, and school performance.[13] Anxiety and depression are also common in adolescents suffering from severe asthma, as well as in their parents.[14] In adults with asthma, QoL is impacted by a combination of coexisting comorbidities, risk factors and health and psychological factors, activity limitation, negative effects on social life and relationships, problems with finding and keeping employment, and reduced productivity.[15]

ATOPIC DERMATITIS AND CHRONIC URTICARIA

AD is a complex, chronic inflammatory skin disorder that is a result of immune dysregulation and skin barrier dysfunction.[16] Symptoms of AD include intense itching and typical eczematous lesions, and the disease often begins early in life. AD is estimated to affect 7% of adults[17] and 13% of children in the United States.[18] By far, the most burdensome symptom of AD is itch, followed by skin changes such as dryness, scaling, redness, and inflammation.[19]

AD can have a significant impact on QoL.[16,20] The impact of AD on QoL can include social impairment, emotional and behavioral problems, and significant psychological problems, including depression, anxiety, and suicidal ideation.[4,20,21] Children and adolescents with AD are more likely to be diagnosed with ADHD, depression, anxiety, and conduct disorder than children without AD.[22,23] Uncontrolled AD can also lead to sleeping problems and significant caregiver burden.[22] Adults with AD are more likely to have depression and anxiety compared with those without AD.[20,23] Further, the mental health burden of AD can be seen regardless of severity of AD.[21]

Chronic spontaneous urticaria (CSU) is a common skin condition that presents with recurrent wheals (or hives) in various body locations for 6 weeks or longer.[24] The wheals, itch, and unpredictable nature of CSU can lead to significant psychological distress. CSU can affect daily activities, including work and school performance, sleep, and social or emotional functioning.[25,26] Patients with CSU have a significantly higher risk of psychiatric disorders such as anxiety and depression compared with the general population.[26]

FOOD ALLERGY

FA is a growing public health burden, with evidence during the last few decades of increasing prevalence.[27] FA is defined as an adverse immune response to food proteins caused by IgE-mediated and non–IgE-mediated mechanisms, which can trigger systemic responses involving the skin, gastrointestinal and respiratory tracts that can be potentially life threatening.[28]

Unlike generalized anxiety, food allergy anxiety (FAA) is typically associated with FA-specific fears and phobias. Although FAA can have positive impacts on allergen avoidance and emergency preparedness, at high levels or when ongoing in nature, FAA can lead to maladaptive and overavoidant behaviors.[29] Those managing FA may also experience posttraumatic stress symptoms due to ongoing challenges and burdens, the unpredictable nature of food allergen exposure, and allergic reactions.[30] FAA is often a motivating factor for allergic patients to seek out FA treatment such as oral immunotherapy due to anxiety about fatal reactions and perceived danger of living with an untreated FA.[31]

FA is a diagnosis that influences family systems, influencing the QoL and anxiety levels of allergic children as well as their parents and caregivers.[32] Common psychosocial burdens affecting individuals and families managing FA include impacts on emotional and physical QoL, daily functioning, social behaviors, and life experiences. Constant stress and vigilance associated with allergen avoidance and potential allergic reactions has an impact on parental mental health and QoL.[33] Additionally, allergy-related bullying is common and associated with lower QoL and distress in allergic children and their parents.[34] Food allergic children and adolescents are twice as likely to be bullied than their nonallergic peers.[35]

Less is known about the burden of FA in the adult population. However, a substantial proportion of food allergic adults do not have a current epinephrine autoinjector prescription, especially if they have adult-onset FA.[36] Many adults report having an FA without proper physician diagnosis, highlighting the importance of appropriate testing to confirm a diagnosis and robust patient education, because unnecessary food avoidance can lead to reduced QoL.

Box 1
Dermatology life quality index[43]

During the last week...
1. How itchy, sore, painful, or stinging has your skin been?
2. How embarrassed or self-conscious have you been because of your skin?
3. How much has your skin interfered with you going shopping or looking after your home?
4. How much has your skin influenced the clothes you wear?
5. How much has your skin affected any social or leisure activities?
6. How much has your skin made it difficult for you to play or do any sport?
7. Has your skin prevented you from working or studying?
8. How much has your skin created problems with your partner, close friends, or relatives?
9. How much has your skin caused any sexual difficulties?
10. How much of a problem has the treatment for your skin been? For example, by taking up time, or being messy?

SCREENING AND MANAGEMENT

Health-care clinicians seeing patients with allergic conditions must be aware of comorbid mental health disorders and the need for social and/or emotional support services.[3,4,37] Health-care clinicians must also be educated on the signs and symptoms of mental health conditions in patients with chronic illness. Detection and treatment can improve control of disease and better adherence to medications.[21] Screening for and addressing these psychiatric comorbidities should be part of patient management.[19,26,38] It is beneficial to evaluate both child and caregiver distress levels and QoL influences and also to provide both with robust education and with referrals to support networks to help reduce the burden FA has on the family system.[39,40] Early recognition and intervention of psychiatric comorbidities can reduce the disease burden.[4,37] Appropriately stepping-up treatment and better control of disease improves mental health and QoL in many patients.[41] In addition to clinical tools to assess symptom burden and control of disease, there are numerous general and disease-specific screening tools that can be used to screen patients who may be at risk for mental health concerns.[42–45] For example, the short form 12 is one of the most widely used screening tools to measure disease-related QoL and can easily be administered in the clinical setting.[42] There are numerous disease-specific QoL questionnaires to help screen for mental health conditions in atopic patients. Some examples include the Dermatology Life Quality Index, which has been shown to correlate with reported pruritus and severity of AD.[43] There are several asthma-specific screening tools, including the Mini Asthma Quality of Life Questionnaire (MiniAQLQ).[44] The Survey of Food Allergy Anxiety is an example of a condition-specific screening tool for pediatric food allergic patients.[45] In the future, depression and anxiety screening should be addressed in guideline updates for allergic conditions.[21] Some of these screening tools are shown in **Boxes 1–3**.

Management includes referral to mental health specialists such as clinical therapists, social workers, psychologists, and psychiatrists to help patients develop an effective balance between emotional distress and QoL. Upon referral, behavioral health-care clinicians provide psychoeducation and use evidence-based modalities including cognitive behavioral therapy to teach coping, self-monitoring, and problem-solving skills.[46] A stepwise approach to assessing for mental health conditions in patients with atopic disease is illustrated in **Fig. 1**.

Box 2
Mini Asthma Quality of Life Questionnaire (MiniAQLQ)[44]

In general, how much of the time during the last 2 weeks (because of your asthma) did you:
1. Feel short of breath?
2. Feel bothered by or had to avoid dust in the environment?
3. Feel frustrated?
4. Feel bothered by coughing?
5. Feel afraid of not having your asthma medication available?
6. Experience a feeling of chest tightness or chest heaviness?
7. Feel bothered by or had to avoid cigarette smoke in the environment?
8. Have difficulty getting a good night's sleep?
9. Feel concerned about having asthma?
10. Experience a wheeze in your chest?
11. Feel bothered by or had to avoid going outside because of weather or air pollution?

How limited have you been during the last 2 weeks doing these activities because of your asthma:
12. Strenuous activities (such as hurrying, exercising, running up stairs, sports)?
13. Moderate activities (such as walking, housework, gardening, shopping, climbing stairs)?
14. Social activities (such as talking, playing with pets/children, visiting friends/relatives)?
15. Work-related activities (tasks you have to do at work)?

Questions are answered on a 7-point scale between All of the time (1 point) and None of the time (7 points).

The score is calculated as the average of domain items and a change in score of greater than 0.5 can be considered clinically important.

Box 3
Survey of Food Allergy Anxiety-Child-Brief[45]

During the last week only, circle the number next to each statement that best describes you:
1. I am scared to eat the food from a new restaurant
2. I try not to be touched by someone because I am scared this will give me an allergic reaction
3. I am scared to eat at parties or the homes of my friends
4. I am scared to eat at the regular lunch table at school or camp
5. I am scared to eat the food served by my school or camp
6. I am too scared to eat food when I am with an adult who is not my parent, like when I am staying with a family member or at a friend's house
7. I am afraid of smelling the foods I am allergic to
8. I am scared to touch safe foods because of the chance of an allergic reaction
9. I am scared that a food I am allergic to will make me very sick if it touches me
10. I am scared to sit next to someone who is eating a food that I am allergic to
11. I am scared to eat safe foods that have been next to foods I am allergic to
12. I check food labels more than I need to because I am scared
13. I ask my parents too many times if a food is safe for me to eat
14. I try not to touch things such as door handles, phones, or clean surfaces because I am afraid of having an FA reaction

Questions are answered on a 5-point scale between Never (0 points) and Almost always (4 points). Add the total score; higher scores indicate greater anxiety.

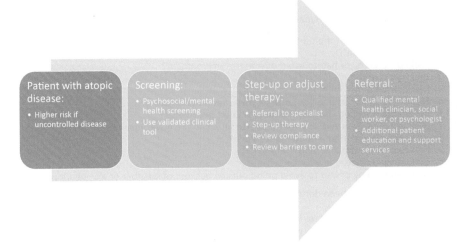

Fig. 1. Simplified, step-wise approach to assessing and managing atopic patients at risk for comorbid mental health conditions.

SUMMARY

Allergic diseases are common and have significant associations with reduced QoL and mental health conditions. There are significant psychosocial burdens facing many patients with atopic conditions, leading to an increased risk of depression, anxiety, emotional and relationship problems, bullying, and sleep disturbances. Clinicians who see patients with allergic conditions must be aware of the increased risk of mental health complications, and appropriately screen patients. There are numerous screening tools available, both general and disease-specific, that can be completed in the clinical setting to help identify patients at risk for mental health conditions. Optimal management of the physical disease, as well as referral to mental health clinicians familiar with chronic disease, is essential to reducing the psychosocial burden for atopic patients.

CLINICS CARE POINTS

- There are significant associations between mental health conditions and reduced QoL in patients with allergic or atopic conditions.
- Clinicians must be aware of the psychosocial impacts of atopic diseases and be able to properly screen and recognize patients at-risk for mental health conditions.
- Optimal management of medical conditions, as well as early intervention of comorbid psychiatric conditions, leads to best outcomes.
- Prompt referral to and management by licensed mental health clinicians is essential for those assessed as at-risk and/or ineffectively managing psychosocial impacts.

DISCLOSURE

A. Michaud has received honoraria from Regeneron, Novartis, and ThermoFisher Diagnostics. T. Hubbard has received honoraria from FARE and Allergy Insider/ThermoFisher Scientific.

REFERENCES

1. Tzeng NS, Chang HA, Chung CH, et al. Increased Risk of Psychiatric Disorders in Allergic Diseases: A Nationwide, Population-Based, Cohort Study. Front Psychiatr 2018;9(133). https://doi.org/10.3389/fpsyt.2018.00133.
2. American Psychiatric Association. (2022). Diagnostic and statistical manual of mental disorders (5th ed., text rev.). https://doi.org/10.1176/appi.books.9780890425787.
3. Blaiss MS, Hammerby E, Robinson S, et al. The burden of allergic rhinitis and allergic rhinoconjunctivitis on adolescents- a literature review. Ann Allergy Asthma Immunol 2018;121:43–52.
4. Hammer-Helmich L, Linneberg A, Obel C, et al. Mental health associations with eczema, asthma and hay fever in children: a cross-sectional survey. BMJ Open 2016;6:e012637.
5. Valls-Mateus M, Marino-Sanchez F, Ruiz-Echevarria K, et al. Nasal obstructive disorders impact health-related quality of life in adolescents with persistent allergic rhinitis: a real-life study. Pediatr Allergy Immunol 2017;19:19.
6. Fokkens WJ, Lund VJ, Mullol J, et al. EPOS 2012: European position paper on rhinosinusitis and nasal polyps 2012. A summary for otorhinolaryngologists. Rhinology 2012;50(1):1–12.
7. Klonaris D, Doulaptsi M, Karatzanis A, et al. Assessing quality of life and burden of disease in chronic rhinosinusitis: a review. Rhinology online 2019;2:6–13.
8. Khan A, Huynh TMT, Vandeplas G, et al. The GALEN rhinosinusitis cohort: chronic rhinosinusitis with nasal polyps affects health-related quality of life. Rhinology 2019;57(5):343–51.
9. Dierick BJH, van der Molen T, Flokstra-de Blok BMJ, et al. Burden and socioeconomics of asthma, allergic rhinitis, atopic dermatitis and food allergy. Expert Rev Pharmacoecon Outcomes Res 2020;20(5):437–53.
10. Coban H, Aydemir Y. The relationship between allergy and asthma control, quality of life, and emotional status in patients with asthma: a cross-sectional study. Allergy Asthma Clin Immunol 2014;10(1):67.
11. Banjari M, Kano Y, Almadani S, et al. The relation between asthma control and quality of life in children. Int J Pediatr 2018;2018:1–6.
12. Trivedi M, Denton E. Asthma in children and adults-what are the differences and what can they tell us about asthma? Front Pediatr 2019;7:256.
13. Kouzegaran S, Samimi P, Ahanchian H, et al. Quality of life in children with asthma versus healthy children. Open Access Maced J Med Sci 2018;6(8):1413–8.
14. Licari A, Ciprandi R, Marseglia G, et al. Anxiety and depression in adolescents with asthma and in their parents: a study in clinical practice. Monaldi Arch Chest Dis 2019;89(3).
15. Stanescu S, Kirby SE, Thomas M, et al. A systematic review of psychological, physical health factors, and quality of life in adult asthma. NPJ Prim Care Respir Med 2019;29(1):37.
16. Oliveira C, Torres T. More than skin deep: the systemic nature of atopic dermatitis. Eur J Dermatol 2019;29(3):250–8.
17. Hua T, Silverberg JI. Atopic dermatitis in US adults: Epidemiology, association with marital status, and atopy. Ann Allergy Asthma Immunol 2018;121(5):622–4.
18. Silverberg JI, Hanifin JM. Adult eczema prevalence and associations with asthma and other health and demographic factors: a US population-based study. J Allergy Clin Immunol 2013;132(5):1132–8.

19. Silverberg JI, Gelfand JM, Margolis DJ, et al. Patient burden and quality of life in atopic dermatitis in US adults: A population-based cross-sectional study. Ann Allergy Asthma Immunol 2018;121(3):340–7.
20. Cheng BT, Silverberg JI. Depression and psychological distress in US adults with atopic dermatitis. Ann Allergy Asthma Immunol 2019;123(2):179–85.
21. Schonmann Y, Mansfield KE, Hayes JF, et al. Atopic Eczema in Adulthood and Risk of Depression and Anxiety: A Population-Based Cohort Study. J Allergy Clin Immunol Pract 2020;8(1):248–57.e16.
22. Yaghmaie P, Koudelka CW, Simpson EL. Mental health comorbidity in patients with atopic dermatitis. J Allergy Clin Immunol 2013;131(2):428–33.
23. Patel KR, Immaneni S, Singam V, et al. Association between atopic dermatitis, depression, and suicidal ideation: A systematic review and meta-analysis. J Am Acad Dermatol 2019;80(2):402–10.
24. Zuberbier T, Aberer W, Asero R, et al. The EAACI/GA^{2}LEN/EDF/WAO guideline for the definition, classification, diagnosis and management of urticaria. Allergy 2018;73(7):1393–414.
25. Jáuregui I, Ortiz de Frutos FJ, Ferrer M, et al. Assessment of severity and quality of life in chronic urticaria. J Investig Allergol Clin Immunol 2014;24(2):80–6.
26. Chu CY, Cho YT, Jiang JH, et al. Patients with chronic urticaria have a higher risk of psychiatric disorders: a population-based study. Br J Dermatol 2020;182(2):335–41.
27. Tang ML, Mullins RJ. Food allergy: is prevalence increasing? Intern Med J 2017;47(3):256–61.
28. Sicherer SH, Sampson HA. 9. Food allergy. J Allergy Clin Immunol 2006;117(2 Suppl Mini-Primer):S470–5.
29. Polloni L, Muraro A. Anxiety and food allergy: A review of the last two decades. Clin Exp Allergy 2020;50(4):420–41.
30. Weiss D, Marsac ML. Coping and posttraumatic stress symptoms in children with food allergies. Ann Allergy Asthma Immunol 2016;117(5):561–2.
31. Dunlop JH, Keet CA. Goals and motivations of families pursuing oral immunotherapy for food allergy. J Allergy Clin Immunol Pract 2019;7(2):662–3.e18.
32. Cummings AJ, Knibb RC, Erlewyn-Lajeunesse M, et al. Management of nut allergy influences quality of life and anxiety in children and their mothers. Pediatr Allergy Immunol 2010;21(4 Pt 1):586–94.
33. Golding MA, Gunnarsson NV, Middelveld R, et al. A scoping review of the caregiver burden of pediatric food allergy. Ann Allergy Asthma Immunol 2021;127(5):536–47.e3.
34. Shemesh E, Annunziato RA, Ambrose MA, et al. Child and parental reports of bullying in a consecutive sample of children with food allergy. Pediatrics 2013;131(1):e10–7.
35. Muraro A, Polloni L, Lazzarotto F, et al. Comparison of bullying of food-allergic versus healthy schoolchildren in Italy. J Allergy Clin Immunol 2014;134(3):749–51.
36. Gupta RS, Warren CM, Smith BM, et al. Prevalence and Severity of Food Allergies Among US Adults. JAMA Netw Open 2019;2(1):e185630.
37. Edvinsson Sollander S, Fabian H, Sarkadi A, et al. Asthma and allergies correlate with mental health problems in preschool children. Acta Paediatr 2021;110(5):1601–9.
38. Maurer M, Weller K, Bindslev-Jensen C, et al. Unmet clinical needs in chronic spontaneous urticaria. A GA^{2}LEN task force report. Allergy 2011;66(3):317–30.

39. Chow C, Pincus DB, Comer JS. Pediatric Food Allergies and Psychosocial Functioning: Examining the Potential Moderating Roles of Maternal Distress and Overprotection. J Pediatr Psychol 2015;40(10):1065–74.

40. Birdi G, Cooke R, Knibb R. Quality of Life, Stress, and Mental Health in Parents of Children with Parentally Diagnosed Food Allergy Compared to Medically Diagnosed and Healthy Controls. J Allergy 2016;2016:1497375.

41. Silverberg JI. Comorbidities and the impact of atopic dermatitis. Ann Allergy Asthma Immunol 2019;123(2):144–51.

42. Ware J Jr, Kosinski M, Keller SD. A 12-Item Short-Form Health Survey: construction of scales and preliminary tests of reliability and validity. Med Care 1996;34(3): 220–33.

43. Finlay AY, Khan GK. Dermatology Life Quality Index (DLQI)–a simple practical measure for routine clinical use. Clin Exp Dermatol 1994;19(3):210–6.

44. Juniper EF, Buist AS, Cox FM, et al. Validation of a standardized version of the Asthma Quality of Life Questionnaire. Chest 1999;115(5):1265–70.

45. Dahlsgaard KK, Wilkey LK, Stites SD, et al. Development of the child- and parent-rated scales of Food Allergy Anxiety (SOFAA). J Allergy Clin Immunol Pract 2022; 10(1):161–9.e6.

46. Herbert L, Shemesh E, Bender B. Clinical management of psychosocial concerns related to food allergy. J Allergy Clin Immunol Pract 2016;4(2):205–13 [quiz: 214].

Office Procedures in the Allergy Practice

David Mangold, BS, MHS, PA-C

KEYWORDS

• Allergy test • Skin test • Prick test • Patch test

KEY POINTS

• Skin prick testing is used to aid in diagnosis of environmental, food, insect, and drug allergies.
• Intradermal allergy testing plays a role primarily in insect and drug allergy testing.
• Patch testing is used to identify contact allergies, primarily for allergic contact dermatitis.

INTRODUCTION

The practicing allergy provider uses many tools to aid in the diagnosis and management of atopic diseases. History taking and physical examination are still extremely important, but what sets an allergy specialist apart is the ability to provide more definitive answers in the office. Without these vital tools, a diagnosis of disease can be made with reasonable accuracy; however, the management and specific recommendations for efficient and effective care require identification of likely allergens and elimination of unlikely ones from treatment plans. To provide appropriate care, diagnostics are essential.

Skin prick testing remains the cornerstone of the initial allergy evaluation for most atopic diseases. It is safe, cost-effective, readily available, rapid, and minimally invasive. For environmental allergens, skin prick testing is often the only tool needed to identify the triggers of disease. For food allergens, it can exclude disease very rapidly so alternative diagnoses can be pursued more rapidly. For stinging insect and drug allergy, it may play an initial role in evaluation of these conditions.

Intradermal skin testing has evolved over the past 2 decades to play less of a role in primary diagnosis of environmental allergies. It still is vital in diagnosing stinging insect and drug allergies. It should not be used for food allergy testing.

Patch testing for contact allergens is the only method of identifying triggers of allergic contact dermatitis. It is an essential tool for anyone evaluating dermatitis patients. Patch testing panels have become better studied and more comprehensive in recent years and thus the likelihood of identifying relevant allergens has increased.

Allergy & Asthma Center, PC, 95 Indian Trail Road, Kalispell, MT 59901, USA
E-mail address: dave@montanaallergy.com

Physician Assist Clin 8 (2023) 695–704
https://doi.org/10.1016/j.cpha.2023.05.005
2405-7991/23/© 2023 Elsevier Inc. All rights reserved.

Patch testing can be time consuming and requires the provider to be adept at providing useful avoidance information once they are completed.

History

The father of skin testing for environmental allergies was Dr. Charles Harrison Blackley from Manchester, England, who identified pollen as the trigger for outdoor environmental allergies in 1873. He isolated pollen as the relevant allergen-causing hay fever and did tests on himself by introducing pollen into his nose, mouth, eyes, and skin. These findings were discussed at length with Charles Darwin who exchanged letters with Dr. Blackley regarding his scientific findings in the newly developed allergy specialty.[1]

The first publication to discuss patch testing for contact allergens was in 1895 by the German Dermatologist, Josef Jadassohn. He placed the suspected allergen on the skin and covered it with an occlusive until a positive result was identified. The technique is largely the same today except the allergens used are now mostly standardized and controlled for non-irritating concentrations.[2]

Definitions

- Scratch test/prick test—Application of a liquid allergen to the superficial dermis using a prick or puncture device to elicit an immediate IgE response with a wheal and flare.
- Intradermal test—Application of aqueous allergen between the dermal layers to raise a bleb to elicit an immediate IgE response with a wheal and flare.
- Patch test—Application of a contact allergen that is non-irritating to the surface of the skin and held in place to elicit a contact reaction in an allergic patient.
- Food allergy—A Type 1, IgE-mediated, immediate, reproducible response involving mast cells to a particular food protein.
- Environmental allergy—A Type 1, IgE-mediated, immediate, reproducible response involving mast cells to a particular airborne allergen (ie, animals, mold, dust mites, pollen).
- Allergic contact dermatitis—A T-cell-mediated, Type 4, delayed immune sensitivity to an allergen that causes a spongiotic dermatitis.

BACKGROUND

The diagnosis of allergic disease can be challenging in the primary care setting. The majority of the diagnosis is based on the patient's history. The first question that needs to be answered is whether the patient's symptoms are truly allergic in nature. Non-allergic rhinitis, other forms of dermatitis, and food intolerances will often be attributed to an "allergy" by the patient. The general public does not typically grasp the difference between an allergic disease and a symptom that seems to be caused by an environmental or food trigger. For example, facial flushing with alcohol can be blamed on an "alcohol allergy" rather than the vasodilation that occurs with alcohol ingestion in some patients. The practicing provider needs to be able to discern between what is truly allergic or not. An improper diagnosis can lead to increased morbidity and decreased quality of life by patients unnecessarily avoiding products that do not need to be avoided.

Another source of confusion lies in the inappropriate use, or improper methods, of allergy testing. Specific IgE testing, whether by serum or with skin tests, remains the best method for identifying allergic triggers of disease. However, even these tests have significant limitations if not interpreted properly in the context of reproducible symptoms. There is no role for any other types of allergy tests in the diagnosis of Type 1 hypersensitivity reactions. Saliva, stool, and hair sample testing is not accurate. IgA, IgG, IgG4, or combined IgE/IgG testing has never been shown to correlate with reproducible allergic disease and should not be used for diagnosis at all.[3] These tests are readily marketed to the general public and alternative health providers, but often just create confusion for the patients when the results do not fit with their history. Even specific IgE tests have high false-positive rates and can be misleading if used as the sole means of diagnosis.

Allergic contact dermatitis is even more challenging to diagnose by history alone. Quite frequently the clinical symptoms will not appear for several days after the allergen exposure. With no treatment, the rash can linger for weeks to months even though there is no continued contact with the allergen. It is also highly likely that the contact allergy is to a product or object that has previously been tolerated. These factors make historical diagnosis almost impossible and extremely frustrating for the patient and provider to figure out without the aid of a diagnostic test. Patch testing for allergic contact dermatitis must also be used in conjunction with history and physical examination. It is common to find positive tests that are not relevant to the patient's environment or pattern of dermatitis.

DISCUSSION: SKIN PRICK TESTING

Skin prick testing is performed by introducing an appropriate concentration of allergen into the superficial dermis to elicit localized mast cell degranulation when specific IgE receptors are bound by the allergen (**Figs. 1-4**). This manifests with a wheal and flare response that can be quantified. The wheal and flare are typically measured at 15 minutes after application. The standard is to measure the wheal and flare in millimeters. Graded scales (1+, 2+, etc) should not be utilized as these are subjective and cannot be interpreted by other providers accurately. Appropriate control tests must be performed to give validity to the skin prick test. A negative control should be utilized to give a baseline wheal and flare response to the skin simply being pricked with the diluent used in the allergy serums. Typically, this will be a solution of human serum albumin with phenol. If a patient has dermatographism then a wheal and flare could be seen to the negative control. The results of the allergen tests should be interpreted based on the value of the negative control. A synthetic histamine control should yield a wheal of at least 3 mm greater than the negative control as well as a corresponding flare. If a positive histamine control is not seen, then the test is deemed inconclusive. This most often occurs if a patient has been using a medication that blocks histamine receptors. There is no need to discontinue steroids or leukotriene receptor antagonists

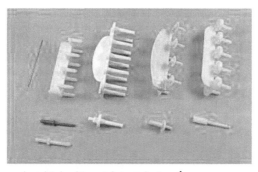

Fig. 1. Some single and multiple skin prick test devices.[4]

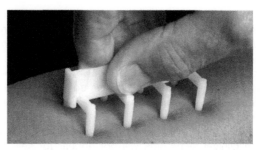

Fig. 2. A multiple test device performing skin prick testing.[6]

prior to skin prick testing. Antihistamine eye drops, nasal sprays, topical creams, or oral formulations should be discontinued for up to a week prior to testing depending on half-life. Tricyclic antidepressants have antihistamine effects and may need to be discontinued for up to 14 days prior to testing. If the patient is unable to discontinue these medications prior to skin testing then consideration for serum-specific IgE testing should be considered. Serum testing does not require discontinuation of medications as the measurement for positivity does not require visualizing an in vitro wheal and flare response.

Skin prick testing has a very low incidence of causing systemic reactions, even in patients who have significant anaphylactic allergies to a substance. The incidence of systemic reaction to skin prick testing has been found to be 0.4%.[5] This low rate of systemic reaction is in part to the use of properly diluted allergens. These appropriate skin test concentrations have been identified and come from commercial suppliers who ensure the testing agent meets quality control standards. There are several different devices that can be utilized for skin prick testing. Some devices contain multiple test heads that allow for testing to a large number of allergens in a rapid manner. Individual devices are also available that allow for more customization of tests, rather than having to test to all components of an allergen panel, including tests that may not be relevant given the patient's history. Regardless of the method or device used, skin prick testing is relatively non-invasive compared with venipuncture and can be accomplished in patients of all ages, including infants.

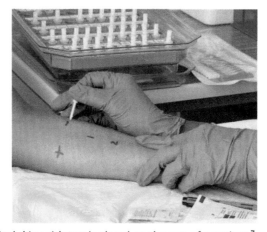

Fig. 3. An individual skin prick test is placed on the arm of a patient.[7]

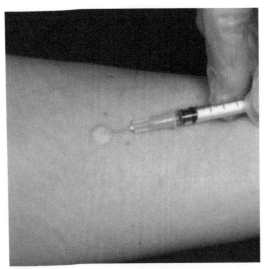

Proper application of an intradermal skin test.[11].

gen extract is injected to raise a bleb. The test is incubated for 15 minutes and the wheal and flare are measured similar to skin prick testing in millimeters, rather n graded scale. Appropriate negative and positive controls are also used to ensure curate skin response. It is essential that the negative control be performed by intra-rmal method using the same diluent the allergenic extracts are diluted in. This is pre critical than in skin prick testing because the blebs that the intradermal test rai-es can be falsely interpreted as a wheal if the negative control is not similar to the test ites. The same medications described above that can interfere with skin prick testing must also be discontinued for intradermal skin testing as they will blunt the wheal and flare response.

Intradermal testing is more invasive that prick testing and elicits much more pain and discomfort. The incidence of systemic reactions is higher at 3.6%.[5] Well established dilutions for many drugs, as well as stinging insect venoms, must be utilized to minimize the chance of systemic reaction. Typically, these tests will start with dilute extracts and then increase in concentration as the testing progresses so a systemic reaction does not occur. The sensitivity and specificity of intradermal testing varies depending on the type of allergen being tested and is difficult to compare, but in general has been shown to be 79.4% and 67.9%, respectively.[12] Appropriate precautions to prevent transmission of bloodborne pathogens and needle sticks should be utilized for any providers performing intradermal testing.

DISCUSSION: PATCH TESTING

Patch testing is currently the only diagnostic test available to identify causative agents in allergic contact dermatitis. Patch testing is not helpful for identifying causes of irritant contact dermatitis. There are no serum tests available for Type IV delayed contact allergy. Patch testing involves applying a small amount of appropriate concentration of allergen directly to the skin and covering with an occlusive. The allergen is typically left in place for 48 hours and then removed. The testing area is observed for an additional 48 hours before reading the test to determine whether dermatitis develops. A common schedule for patch testing consists of placing the patches on Monday, removing them

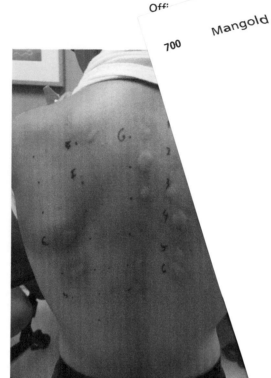

Fig. 4. Typical layout of skin prick tests on patient's back with multiple ~~~

Fig. 5

Skin prick testing is most commonly utilized for evaluation of en~~~
food allergens. The most common environmental allergens would ~~~
mold, animal dander, cockroach, grass, weeds, and trees. The sensiti~~~
ficity for skin prick tests to environmental allergens ranges from 85% to ~~~
to 86%, respectively.[8] Food allergy testing is typically accomplished w~~~
commercially prepared extracts; however, there are some allergens w~~~
made extracts in the allergy office can yield more accurate results. This~~~
some commercially prepared extracts undergo protein denaturization t~~~
sterilization process. The sensitivity and specificity of skin prick testing to ~~~
gens is 85% and 74%, respectively.[9] The sensitivity and specificity for food~~~
cannot be generalized, however, and different cut off points for positive tests~~~
needed for each allergen. For this reason, all patients with positive food allerg~~~
and no clear history of immediate reactivity to the positive foods must be cou~~~
about the high false-positive rate so they are not misled into thinking they have~~~
allergies, unless corroborated with controlled dietary challenges.

DISCUSSION: INTRADERMAL SKIN TESTING

Intradermal skin testing has fallen out of routine use for environmental allergy testin~~~
over the past 2 decades due to high false-positive rates as well as significant discomfort and poor patient satisfaction (**Fig. 5**). Intradermal allergy testing still has appropriate utility for aiding in the diagnosis of drug and stinging insect allergy.
Intradermal skin testing plays no role in diagnosis of food allergy. Intradermal testing
is typically accomplished using tuberculin syringes with 25 to 30 gauge needles. The
needle is inserted between the dermal layers and 0.05 mL of appropriately diluted

on Wednesday, and performing the final reading on Friday. This can prove difficult for patients who live in rural regions and have to drive great distances to have patch testing done. The tests are graded on a standardized scale with the following accepted interpretations: NR = No Reaction, ? = Doubtful Reaction, 1+ = Erythema and Edema, 2+ = Papule Formation, 3+ = Bullous Reaction (**Fig. 6**).

Selection of appropriate patch tests is important. In the United States only the True Test product is FDA approved. The currently available True Test panel tests for 36 allergens. The American Contact Dermatitis Society recommends a panel of 80 to 100 allergens as their core panel to properly screening for allergic contact dermatitis.[14] This panel of core allergens is constantly being reviewed and upgraded based on cosmetic industry trends as well as data from patch testing centers on relevant positive responses. Materials and allergens are available from several other manufacturers to test for these expanded panels beyond True Test. Patch testing can help shorten the time to achieve a final diagnosis from an average of 175 days to an average of 8 days. A final diagnosis is made in 88% of patients who have patch testing compared with 69% of patients who do not have patch testing.[15] Occasionally patch tests can be performed to products or objects the patient brings from home. This should be avoided unless control tests are performed on a healthy subject in the office to ensure that the product is not simply an irritant.

Patch testing is much more technically and logistically challenging than skin prick or intradermal testing for other allergic diseases. Patch testing is usually performed by allergy or dermatology clinics that specialize in contact dermatitis. Patch testing is essential for identifying relevant occupational exposures causing dermatitis. There may also be a role in the use of patch tests for identifying allergens in implantable orthopedic hardware, dental materials, and cardiac devices and stents. Tests for these materials are controversial in clinical relevance and must be part of a shared decision-making discussion between the patient and their other specialty providers (**Fig. 7**).

Patch testing should not be performed if the patient has significantly inflamed skin; however, immune modulators and steroids used to treat dermatitis will interfere with patch test results and could yield false negatives if used within 3 to 4 weeks of the

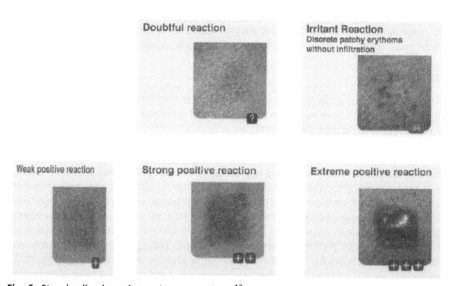

Fig. 6. Standardized patch test interpretations.[13].

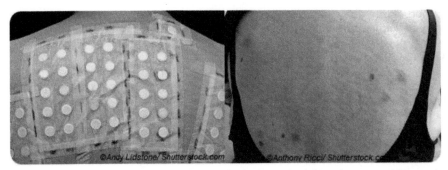

Fig. 7. An example of patch tests applied to the back on the left and some positive results on the right.[16]

patch testing. For patients with persistent, diffuse dermatitis finding a window of clarity in which to perform patch testing is challenging. Antihistamines can be used without interfering with patch tests, but are rarely useful in treating patients with allergic contact dermatitis.

The most important part of patch testing is educating and counseling the patient once the results are available. Allergens that are identified may or may not be relevant to the presenting complaint. Providing a patient with a long list of chemical names to avoid is not typically practical or useful as many of these allergens may go by other chemical names on ingredient lists. It is this author's experience that most patients who find patch testing unhelpful in their diagnostics have been provided information after patch testing that does not allow for successful avoidance measures to be undertaken. The use of the Contact Allergen Management Program (CAMP) through the American Contact Dermatitis Society is an extremely useful tool that is essential to providing accurate and helpful information to patients with positive patch tests.[17] This program allows a user to enter the positive allergens and then select categories of products, such as shampoo, makeup, and laundry detergent. The results of the search include brand names of products that are safe for the patient to use and do not contain relevant allergens. This way a patient never has to read an ingredient list, they simply purchase product names that are given on their handout. The CAMP information is available to the patient by printout, website, or mobile app.

SUMMARY

Allergy testing is an essential tool that aids in the proper diagnosis and treatment of allergic diseases. Proper selection and interpretation of the allergy test is critical. Allergy testing should not be undertaken unless appropriate clinical suspicion for allergic disease is present. This can only be determined by a thorough history and physical examination. If allergy testing is performed with a low clinical suspicion, then the results can be misleading and send the practitioner down treatment pathways that are inappropriate or ineffective at best and potentially harmful at worst. Patients will often want positive allergy tests to provide answers that explain their symptoms. The scientifically inquisitive medical provider will use these tests to not only diagnose allergic disease and identify relevant allergens, but also to rule out allergens that are not part of the patient's problem. Telling a patient, they are not allergic to items allows for opportunities to better identify what the underlying medical issue truly is. The practicing allergy provider must not only be a clinical scientist, but also a comprehensive patient educator. It is important to validate the patient's complaints, investigate their concerns, and educate them on the results of appropriately performed allergy tests.

CLINICS CARE POINTS

- The diagnosis of Type I, IgE-mediated allergy and Type 4, allergic contact dermatitis must be made in conjunction with proper history, physical examination, and appropriate allergy tests, interpreted correctly.

- Not all symptoms that seem allergic to patients and providers are actually allergic diseases. Appropriate allergy testing can help make a correct diagnosis and thus proper treatment can be recommended.

- There are many alternative forms of "allergy tests" in use today for identifying food and environmental allergens, but the only tests that are clinically validated to aid in the diagnosis of allergic disease are specific IgE tests (serum or skin tests).

- Patch testing is an essential tool for identification of relevant allergens that may be causing allergic contact dermatitis. Patch testing should be considered for anyone with persistent dermatitis where an underlying cause cannot be identified through other means.

- Patch testing results must be interpreted accurately and patient education materials must be provided that are useful to the patient and give them tools to help avoid relevant allergens.

DISCLOSURE

The author does not currently have any financial disclosures that are relevant to the topic of allergy testing protocols. The author does not have any commercial conflicts on this topic. The author is a member of the Association of Physician Assistants in Allergy, Asthma and Immunology, American Contact Dermatitis Society, American Academy of Allergy, Asthma and Immunology, as well as a member of the American College of Allergy, Asthma and Immunology.

REFERENCES

1. https://www.darwinproject.ac.uk/charles-harrison-blackley, University of Cambridge.
2. Bernstein L, Li J, Bernstein D, et al. Allergy Diagnostic Testing: An Updated Practice Parameter. Ann Allergy Asthma Immunol 2008;100:S37.
3. Bernstein L, Li J, Bernstein D, et al. Allergy Diagnostic Testing: An Updated Practice Parameter. Ann Allergy Asthma Immunol 2008;100(S4):S10–1.
4. Available at: https://www.jaci-inpractice.org/cms/attachment/2039956669/2053505335/gr2.jpg
5. Bagg A, Chacko T, Lockey R. Reactions to prick and intradermal skin tests. Ann Allergy Asthma Immunol 2009 May;102(5):400–2.
6. Available at: https://media.snacksafely.com/wp-content/uploads/2020/11/Skin-Prick-Testing-1068x559.jpg
7. Available at: https://www.verywellhealth.com/thmb/2mXzJ6jJEzejROGQSC_L2m1iCj8=/1890x1589/filters:fill(87E3EF,1)/GettyImages-544541817-56975a055f9b58eba49e5a00.jpg
8. Bernstein L, Li J, Bernstein D, et al. Allergy Diagnostic Testing: An Updated Practice Parameter. Ann Allergy Asthma Immunol 2008 Mar;100:S20.
9. Sampson H, Aceves S, Bock A. Food allergy: A practice parameter update—2014. J Allergy Clin Immunol 2014. pg. 10.e19.

10. Available at: http://thewalkingallergy.com/wp-content/uploads/2017/07/img_2023.jpg
11. Available at: https://drhuiallergist.com/wp-content/uploads/2015/12/intradermal_skin_test-e1388539484334-300x300.jpg
12. Bernstein L, Li J, Bernstein D, et al. Allergy Diagnostic Testing: An Updated Practice Parameter. Ann Allergy Asthma Immunol 2008 Mar;100:S24.
13. Available at: https://image.slidesharecdn.com/delayedtypedrughypersensitivity interhospitalconference-100803104905-phpapp01/95/delayed-type-drug-hyper sensitivity-46-728.jpg?cb=1280833217
14. Schalock P, Dunnick C, Nedorost S. American Contact Dermatitis Society Core Allergen Series: 2020 Update. Dermatitis 2020;31.
15. Spiewak R. Patch Testing for Contact Allergy and Allergic Contact Dermatitis. Open Allergy J 2008;1:42–51.
16. Available at: https://www.news-medical.net/image.axd?picture=patch%20test_thumb.jpg
17. Available at: http://www.acdscamp.org/

The Diagnosis and Treatment of Atopic Dermatitis

Keri Holyoak, MPH, MSHS, PA-C

KEYWORDS

- Atopic dermatitis • Eczema • Pruritis • Chronic • Inflammation • Lichenification

KEY POINTS

- AD is a challenging inflammatory skin condition with a significant burden on the quality of life.
- Chronic, relapsing cycles of intense itch and erythema is the hallmark of AD.
- New understanding of AD and innovative therapies hold promise for achieving disease control, including in patients with recalcitrant disease.

INTRODUCTION

AD, also known as eczema, is a common inflammatory skin disorder that pervades all cultures and ages.[1,2] Globally, it is the most common chronic skin disease that affects up to 20% of children and 10% of adults.[3,4] 230 million people worldwide are estimated to have AD, with reports that it has the highest disease burden of non-fatal skin disorders.[3]

While the onset of AD typically occurs in the first three to six months after birth, 60% of cases will manifest in the first year and up to 90% by the fifth year.[5,6] It cannot be predicted whether a patient will outgrow their condition and 30% of children continue to have lifelong relapses.[7] Research also suggests that the incidence of AD is increasing in adults between 20 and 40 years old.[8,9] Mohn and colleagues[10] speculate that the rise may be explained by environmental and lifestyle changes in genetically predisposed individuals. Arguable reasons include air pollution, proximity to traffic, increased water hardness, exposure to tobacco smoke, molds, dust mites, animal dander, use of fragranced lotions, and psychological stress.

It is often associated with a personal or family history of atopy, which describes a group of disorders that include food allergies, asthma, and allergic rhinitis.[5] Baseline

The Dermatology Center of Salt Lake, 7396 South Union Park Avenue Suite 201, Midvale, UT 84047, USA
E-mail address: kholyoak@gmail.com

Physician Assist Clin 8 (2023) 705–715
https://doi.org/10.1016/j.cpha.2023.05.006
2405-7991/23/© 2023 Elsevier Inc. All rights reserved.

AD severity is the strongest predictor of persistent AD, and those with a persistent disease commonly noted early involvement in the hands, head, and posterior neck.[11]

BURDEN OF DISEASE

AD adversely and overwhelmingly affects the quality of life of patients, their families, and caregivers. When a child is in a flare, many nights of sleep are lost from parents trying to relieve their child's discomfort and unrelenting itch. Long bedtime and bath routines to apply topical moisturizers and medications occur. In adults, AD can have detrimental effects on patients' health-related quality of life (HRQoL) and adults with mild disease found no differences in patient-reported HRQoL outcomes compared to adults with moderate to severe disease.[12] Patients experience an inability to focus due to the pruritis, decreased self-esteem, depression, difficulties with social activities, impairment in school, and work performance. It can cause irritability, isolation, and carries a significant morbidity and burden. Most patients report itch and sleep disturbances as the most burdensome symptoms and the majority report that their AD as inadequately controlled.[13,14]

CLINICAL FEATURES

AD is difficult to diagnose because of the variable clinical presentation. Severity is determined by the extent of erythema, degree of excoriation, lichenification, intensity of itch, and impact on sleep and daily activities.[15]

The diagnosis is clinical and based heavily on the medical history and physical examination. To aid diagnosis, several sets of criteria have been developed; the most widely cited being the "Hanifin and Rajka" criteria and subsequent modifications, including the UK Working Party's Diagnostic Criteria for Atopic Dermatitis, and the American Academy of Dermatology 2014 Guidelines. Five major clinical features based on these criteria are: (1) pruritus; (2) a chronic, relapsing course; (3) typical distribution; (4) family or personal history of atopy; (5) onset before 2 years of age.

Pruritus is universal and xerosis is a common feature characterized by fine scaling and roughness of the skin. Ill-defined erythematous papules, plaques, excoriations, and serous exudate characterize acute lesions. Extensive scratching of chronic lesions result in thickened, lichenified, hyperpigmented plaques and fibrotic papules.

Infants (birth to 6 months) usually present with facial, scalp, trunk, and extensor surface of extremities usually sparing the diaper area. Truncal lesions are usually ill-defined while lesions on the limbs can be localized.

In young children (6 months to 12 years) lesions have flexural involvement, including the antecubital fossa, popliteal fossa, wrists, ankles, hands, dorsum of feet, and neck. Dennie-Morgan lines or swelling in periorbital skin, indicate active facial AD. As chronic lesions resolve hypopigmentation or hyperpigmentation commonly occurs.

Adolescents (older than 12 years) have diffuse eczema with localized lesions affecting the face, especially the perioral or periorbital areas, flexural areas, hands, and upper trunk.

Adult AD can present with generalized, diffuse erythema with crusted, oozing lesions. Lesions can also be localized predominantly to hands, head (upper lip and eyelid), neck, upper trunk and shoulders, and flexural areas (**Figs. 1–3**). Labial and nipple eczema can been seen in females. Nummular eczema or round, erythematous lesions that can occur on the legs or arms are often refractory to treatment. Patients with long-standing AD experience multiple areas of lichenification and indurated or prurigo nodules.

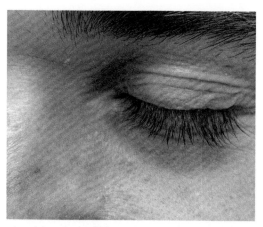

Fig. 1. Scaly plaques involving the eyelid.

Asian or African patients can present with follicular papules, papular lichenoid lesions, palmar hyperlinearity, orbital darkening, and ichthyosis. Erythema in darker skin appears violaceous or may be completely missed in AD.

ADDITIONAL TESTING

There is no specific test used to diagnose AD and a skin biopsy does not assist in differentiating the various forms of AD in adults. Serum IgE is the most common

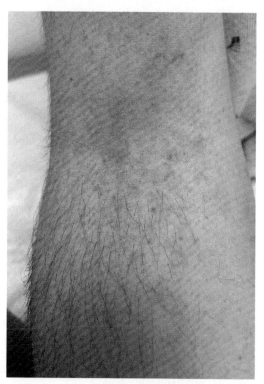

Fig. 2. Erythematous plaques with fine scale and excoriations at the antecubital fossa.

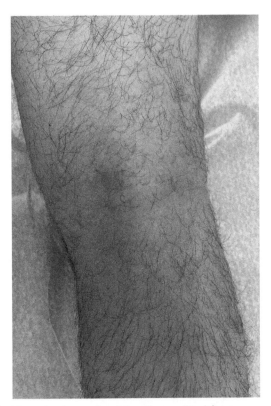

Fig. 3. Ill-defined, thin scaly plaques involving the popliteal fossa.

laboratory finding, but is not recommended for monitoring disease severity because IgE is not present in approximately 20% of patients with AD and some develop elevated IgE levels later in the course of the disease.[5] Skin patch testing is the gold standard for identifying contact allergies.[16] It is most useful when diagnosing adults if the history suggests an exposure to a possible allergen, in chronic AD not responding to appropriate treatment or when the pattern of AD is atypical and changing.[17]

PATHOPHYSIOLOGY

The pathogenesis of AD is complex and consists of multiple interactions between immunological disturbances, a dysfunctional epidermal barrier, and skin microbiome abnormalities. It also depends on genetic, environmental, and personal factors.

Genetic factors are important contributors in AD and a family history of atopic disease is a risk factor. If one parent is atopic, there is more than a 50% chance that their offspring will develop atopic symptoms. If both parents are affected, up to 80% of children will be affected.[18] Other genetic alterations include a change in the function of the gene encoding the synthesis of filaggrin (FLG), an essential epidermal protein that has a pivotal role in maintaining the integrity of the epidermal barrier in the keratinocytes. Impaired filaggrin synthesis leads to increased transepidermal water loss (TEWL) and an increased risk of environmental antigens entering the skin. Filaggrin mutations are present in up to 30% of patients with AD and may also predispose patients to ichthyosis vulgaris, allergic rhinitis, and keratosis pilaris.

Environmental factors are individual and include non-specific factors such as airborne irritants, exposures to soaps, detergents, or fragranced fabric softeners, sweating, and heat. Tight-fitting clothing, rough fabrics such as wool and acrylics, seasonal changes in temperature, or humidity and exposure to wet/irritating substances may also play a role.

An inherited dysfunctional skin barrier is a hallmark factor in the pathogenesis of AD as shown by elevated TEWL, pH, increased permeability, and tears of AD skin. The integrity of the skin barrier is further lost when physical damage occurs from scratching and by microbial dysbiosis, including the colonization of S. aureus and cutaneous yeasts such as Malassezia species. Approximately 90% of patients with AD experience S. aureus colonization and up to 50%–60% of the colonizing S. aureus is toxin-producing causing damage to the protective skin barrier allowing for entry of invading allergens and pathogens that further drive the pathogenesis of AD.[19,20] As a result, patients produce an increased amount of pro-allergic cytokines, such as interleukin-4 (IL-4), IL-5, and IL-13. These cytokines lead to an increased infiltration of inflammatory T cells and eosinophils. IL-4 and IL-13 also are important for the production of serum IgE, the level of which can be elevated in patients with AD. IL-4 and IL-13 mediate downstream signal transduction to suppress the innate immune response genes, thereby making patients with AD more susceptible to skin infections with herpes simplex virus and S. aureus.[19]

Immunological dysregulation and inflammation via an overactive Th2 immune response are central to the pathogenesis of AD. This results in the production of Th2-mediated cytokines, leading to increased IL-4, IL-13, IL-22, and IL-31 (the so-called "pruritis cytokine"), and plasma synthesis of IgE through the signal transducer and activator of transcription (STAT) pathway.[21] Th17, Th22, and Th1 cytokines are also involved depending on the phase of AD, patient age and ethnic background.[22] In patients of Asian decent an activation of Th1-mediated and Th17-mediated responses have been reported but the importance of this pathway is unclear and inhibition of these do not appear to be an effective therapeutic intervention for AD.[23] Knowing the immunotype of the patients with AD, therapeutic plans may be more precise in future treatment plans.

The itch of AD is induced by a complex variety of pruritogens. As patients itch, they further damage the skin barrier, allowing allergens and irritants to enter the epidermis, and activate signals that perpetuate the itch-scratch cycle. Histamine is an important pruritogen released from mast cells and basophils. However, there is no evidence that antihistamines are effective improving signs and symptoms of AD, including itch.[24] Several type 2 immune cells release IL-31, which drives itch even more. Other type 2 cytokines, including IL-4, IL-13, thymic stromal lymphopoietin (TSLP), and IL-31, contribute to itch and might be more relevant to chronic pruritis in AD.

Lesional AD skin shows dysregulated expression of several genes, mostly related to keratinocyte activity and T-cell infiltration, especially for Th2-associated (IL-4, IL-10, IL-13) and Th22-associated (IL-22) genes. Reduced natural killer (NK) cell-mediated immunomodulation has also been considered to be involved in the immune dysregulation in AD. Decreased concentration and altered composition of peripheral blood NK cells, and enrichment of lesional skin with activated NK cells might serve as potential counter-regulatory responses to inflammation.[25]

The janus kinase (JAK)- STAT pathway has effects on the regulation of Th2 differentiation, signaling downstream of cytokines such as IL-4, IL-5, and IL-13, and plays another role in AD. Activation of JAK is followed by the phosphorylation of STAT, which in its active state translocates to the cell nucleus for gene transcription. Studies have shown the JAK-STAT pathways are involved in mediating the inflammation process, changes of natural skin barriers, and increased TEWL by interactions of a number of cytokines causing AD.[20]

TREATMENT

Treatment of AD is long-term and aims to improve and manage itch, clear existing lesions and establish disease control. A patient-centered, step-up, and step-down management approach for acute flares and chronic disease is essential. Educating patients, families, and caregivers on AD improves disease severity and quality of life.

Regardless of severity, all patients with AD need education on basic skin care, including the use of moisturizers to increase skin hydration, bathing, and trigger avoidance. Moisturizers should have few ingredients, without fragrances, or preservatives to avoid irritants and allergic reactions and should be applied every 4 hours to all skin, even uninvolved areas. In general, plain petrolatum can be used if contact dermatitis resulting from additives in medication is suspected.

Application of a moisturizer after regular, 10-minute lukewarm baths help prevent TEWL and hydrate the skin. Soap, bubble baths, and shower gels should be avoided along with washcloths and brushes to cleanse the skin. A randomized trial found no evidence for bath additives, including bath oils, oatmeal, or baking soda effective for the relief of skin irritation and pruritis.[26,27]

Supplementation of vitamin D can be considered a safe and tolerable therapy that may have a beneficial effect in AD. While the data may be conflicting, the majority of studies suggest that vitamin D is protective against AD.[28] In addition, meta-analyses have shown that vitamin D supplementation results in an improvement in AD severity in two clinical tools, scoring AD (SCORAD) and eczema area and severity index (EASI), used for assessing the severity of AD as objectively as possible.[29]

Topical corticosteroids (TCS) are endorsed when basic skin management alone does not control disease. The lowest potency of TCS that is effective should be used and only for short periods due to local side effects, including tachyphylaxis, ski atrophy, purpura, striae, telangiectasias, dyspigmentation, and acneiform changes. Hypothalamic-pituitary-adrenal suppression and growth suppression are considered very uncommon systemic side effects from topical corticosteroids. The choice of the TCS is based on severity of disease, patient age, and disease location. Milder disease, younger age, and flexural and facial skin involvement are reasons to use a less potent TCS, except in cases of a severe flare.

Low potency TCSs include classes V to VII (dexamethasone 0.1% cream, desonide 0.05%, hydrocortisone butyrate 0.1%) can be applied twice a day, including on the face, for two weeks. Medium potency TCS includes class III or IV (triamcinolone acetonide 0.1%, mometasone furoate 0.1% cream) can be applied twice a day for two weeks. High potency includes class II or I (clobetasol propionate or halobetasol propionate) can be applied twice a day for two weeks.

Topical calcineurin inhibitors (TCIs), including tacrolimus (protopic) and pimecrolimus (elidel) have steroid-like anti-inflammatory effects, with no skin atrophy, can be used in areas such as the face, skin folds, and genitals. Stinging and burning are commonly experienced with their use and the high cost restricts their use. TCIs are recommended when TCS fail or are contraindicated. They are not indicated for children less than two years of age.

A wet-wrap dressing is a technique that can be used after emollients and can be beneficial in cases of exacerbated skin lesions. Dampened cotton garments or a towel may be worn over the affected area and covered with a dry garment twice a day for 15 minutes over a five-day period. These reduce TEWL, soothe and hydrate the skin, reduce itching and redness, loosen crusted areas, prevent skin injury due to scratching, and improve the efficacy of the emollient.[30]

Dilute bleach baths, twice weekly, can be used in patients with recurrent skin infections. One-fourth cup of regular, unconcentrated household bleach (5.25% sodium hyperchlorite) added to a 20-gallon bath can reduce the risk of infections and manage eczema flares. Long-term use of a topical antibiotic is not recommended as it can cause resistant microbiome on the skin.

Crisaborole ointment, a topical inhibitor of the intracellular enzyme phosphodiesterase-4 (PDE-4), is a topical non-steroid option for patients with mild-to-moderate AD as young as 3 months old. PDE-4 is an enzyme inside cells that produces cytokines. Blocking PDE-4 hinders the production of several cytokines that are involved in AD. It can be used in sensitive or non-sensitive sites twice a day.

Topical JAK inhibitors can penetrate through the skin due to their small molecular size. Ruxolitinib (opzelura) 1.5% cream is a selective JAK1 and JAK2 inhibitor indicated for mild to moderate AD in non-immunocompromised patients 12 years and older. In 2 identical phase 3 double-blind, randomized, vehicle-controlled trials on 1249 adult and adolescent patients aged 12 years or older with mild to moderate AD 53.8% versus 15.1% vehicle and 51.3% versus 7.6% vehicle achieved clear or almost clear skin by week 8.[31] It can be used twice a day up to 8 weeks for prompt antipruritic effects.

If AD cannot be controlled topically, narrowband ultraviolet B light therapy (nbUVB) and medium dose ultraviolet A1 can be used.[32] Phototherapy is expensive, and may increase the risk of skin cancer, and is therefore recommended only for people with severe eczema whose symptoms do not respond to other treatments.

Systemic Treatments

The most common systemic treatments for AD include cyclosporin, methotrexate, azathioprine, and mycophenolate mofetil. However, their use is limited by long-term toxicity. Robust long-term data on the effects of these drugs in AD are largely missing, and most trials remain placebo controlled with no head-to-head comparisons.[33] Oral steroids, such as prednisone, may be used in acute, severe exacerbations and as a short-term bridge to other systemic, steroid-sparing therapy. However, after stopping an oral steroid a "rebound effect" can occur whereby the symptoms of AD return, often worse.

Biologics

Dupilumab (dupixent) a fully human monoclonal antibody against the IL-4 and IL-13 receptors is approved in adults and children 6 months of age and older. It is the first biologic approved for moderate to severe AD. In two phase 3 monotherapy randomized trials in adults, 51.3% and 44.2% of patients who received dupilumab 300 mg every other week achieved a 75% improvement from baseline an (EASI 75) at week 16, compared with 14.7% and 25% in placebo groups.[34] When combined with topical corticosteroids, the proportion of patients achieving an EASI75 response increased to approximately 65% compared with 22% for topical corticosteroids only and response rates were sustained until week 52.[35] Dupilumab has a tolerable safety profile, including transitory conjunctivitis that can be managed with topical anti-inflammatory ocular agents, being the most frequent side effect observed in dupilumab users.[36]

Tralokinumab-ldrm (adbry), a biologic specifically targeting IL-13 for adults, was approved in 2022 for moderate to severe AD. Phase 3 randomized, double-blind, placebo-controlled trials, included 2,000 adult patients with moderate to severe AD. At week 16, 16% and 21% of patients treated with adbry 300 mg every other week achieved clear or almost clear skin (Investigator Global Assessment 0/1) versus 7% and 9% with placebo.[37]

Many other agents, such as lebrikizumab, tralokinumab and nemolizumab, as well as antibodies against OX40, IL-22, and IL-17 are in clinical investigation. This may expand the range of biologic therapies in the future.[38]

Oral Janus Kinase Inhibitors

JAKs are intracellular enzymes that mediate the signaling cascade from a cytokine receptor in the cell. The JAK family has 4 members: JAK1, JAK2, JAK3, and tyrosine kinase (TYK2). JAK inhibitors can target one or more of these family members to hinder their effects, leading to improvement in signs and symptoms of AD. The first oral JAK1 inhibitors approved in the United States are abrocitinib and upadacitinib. There is a boxed warning for all JAK inhibitors, regarding the risk of serious infections, mortality, malignancy, major cardiovascular events, and thrombosis.

Abrocitinib (cibinqo) is approved for adults 18 years and older with moderate to severe AD. Phase 3, randomized, placebo-controlled clinical trials were designed to evaluate the efficacy and safety of 2 doses (100 mg and 200 mg once daily) with primary endpoints and EASI75 responses. At week 12, 23.7% of patients given abrocitinib 100 mg and 43.8% of patients given abrocitinib 200 mg achieved clear or almost clear skin (IGA 0/1) vs. 8% with placebo.[39] 39.7% (100 mg) and 62.7% (200 mg) achieved an EASI 75 compared to 17.9% and 11.8% in the placebo group. Nausea, headache, and nasopharyngitis are the most frequently reported adverse events. There were also transient dose-related decreases in median platelet count and a higher incidence of herpes zoster and simplex, likely an outcome common to all JAK inhibitors.[39]

Upadacitinib (rinvoq) is approved for adults and children 12 years and older with refractory, moderate to severe atopic dermatitis. Approval of 2 dose strengths (15 mg and 30 mg) was supported by efficacy and safety data from one of the largest Phase 3 programs in AD with more than 2,500 patients evaluated. Rinvoq demonstrated significantly higher levels of skin clearance (EASI 90 and EASI 100) at 16 weeks, compared to placebo.[40] Acne, creatinine phosphokinase elevation, and nasopharingitis were the most frequently reported adverse events.[41]

SUMMARY

AD is a challenging chronic skin condition. It has a complex etiology including genetic and environmental factors, which lead to abnormalities in the epidermis and the immune system. Visible erythematous, scaling, lichenified skin with oozing sores can exacerbate the stigma and contribute to adverse psychosocial and health outcomes. There is legitimate hope to decrease the burden for this challenging condition with new understanding of AD pathogenesis and novel, targeted therapeutic treatments.

CLINICS CARE POINTS

- Treatment of AD is long-term and aims to improve and manage itch, clear existing lesions and establish disease control.
- Regardless of severity, all patients with AD need education on basic skin care, including the use of moisturizers to increase skin hydration, bathing, and trigger avoidance.

DISCLOSURE

The author has no relevant financial interests to declare.

REFERENCES

1. Sandeep K, Watson W, Carr S. Atopic dermatitis. Allergy Asthma Clin Immunol 2018;14(2):44–52.
2. Weidinger S, Beck L, Bieber T. Atopic dermatitis. Nat Rev Dis Primers 2018; 4(1):1–20.
3. Langan S, Irvine A, Weidinger S. Atopic Dermatitis. Lancet 2020;396:345–60.
4. Archer C. Atopic eczema. Medicine (Abingdon) 2013;41(6):341–4.
5. Eichenfield L, Tom W, Chamlin S, et al. Guidelines of care for the management of atopic dermatitis: section 1. Diagnosis and assessment of atopic dermatitis. J Am Acad Dermatol 2014;70(2):338–51.
6. Williams H. Clinical practice. Atopic dermatitis. N Engl J Med 2005;352(22): 2314–415.
7. Ozkaya E. Adult-onset atopic dermatitis. J Am Acad Dermatol 2005;52(4): 579–82.
8. Laughter M, Maymone M, Mashayekhi S, et al. The global burden of disease of atopic dermatitis from 1990–2017. Br J Dermatol 2021;184(2):E42.
9. Kim J, Chao L, Simpson E, et al. Persistence of atopic dermatitis (AD): a systemic review and meta-analysis. J Am Acad Dermatol 2016;75(4):681–7.e11.
10. Mohn C, Blix H, Halvorsen J, et al. Incidence trends of atopic dermatitis in infancy and early childhood in a nationwide prescription registry study in norway. JAMA Netw Open 2018;1(7):e184145.
11. Chovatiya R, Silverberg J. Evaluating the longitudinal course of atopic dermatitis: a review of the literature. J Am Acad Dermatol 2022. Available at: https://www. sciencedirect.com/science/article/pii/S0190962222002535. Accessed March 9, 2022.
12. Whiteley J, Emir B, Seitzman R, et al. The burden of atopic dermatitis in US adults: results from the 2013 National Health and Wellness Survey. Curr Med Res Opin 2016;32(10):1645–51.
13. Wenhui W, Anderson P, Gadhari A. Extent and consequences of inadequate disease control among adults with a history of moderate to severe atopic dermatitis. J Dermatol 2018;45(2):150–7.
14. Silverberg J, Gelfand J, Margolis D, et al. Patient burden and quality of life in atopic dermatitis in US adults: a population based cross-sectional study. Ann Allergy Asthma Immunol 2018;121(3):340–7.
15. Lio P, Lee M, LeBovidge J, et al. Clinical management of atopic dermatitis: practical highlights and updates from the Atopic Dermatitis Practice Parameter 2012. J Allergy Clin Immunol Pract 2014;2(4):361–9.
16. Barrett M, Luu M. Differential diagnosis of atopic dermatitis. Immunol Allergy Clin N Am 2017;37(1):11–34.
17. Silvestre Salvador J, Romero-Perez D, Encabo-Duran B. Atopic dermatitis in adults: a diagnostic challenge. J Investig Allergol Clin Immunol 2017;27(2): 78–88.
18. Kolb L, Ferrer-Bruker S. Atopic Dermatitis. Available at: https://www.ncbi.nlm.nih. gov/books/NBK448071/. Accessed on March 15, 2022.
19. Park K, Pak S, Park K. The pathogenetic effect of natural and bacterial toxins on atopic dermatitis. Toxins 2016;9(1):3.

20. Krzysztof S, Trzeciak M, Nowicki R. Review JAK-STAT inhibitors in atopic dermatitis from pathogenesis to clinical trials results. Microorganisms 2020;8(11):1743.

21. Gittler J, Shemer A, Suarez-Farinas M, et al. Progressive activation of T(H)2/T(H)22 cytokines and selective epidermal proteins characterizes acute and chronic atopic dermatitis. J Allergy Clin Immunol 2012;130:1344–54.

22. Khattri S, Brunner P, Garcet S, et al. Efficacy and safety of ustekinumab treatment in adults with moderate-to-severe atopic dermatitis. Exp Dermatol 2017;177:419–27.

23. Saeki H, Kabashima K, Tokura Y, et al. Efficacy and safety of ustekinuman in Japanese patients with severe atopic dermatitis: a randomized, double-blind, placebo-controlled, phase II study. Br J Dermatol 2017;177:419–27.

24. Matterne U, Bohmer M, Weisshaar E, et al. Oral H1 antihistamines as "add-on' therapy to topical treatment for eczema. Cochrane Database Syst Rev 2019;1: CD012167.

25. Mack M, Brestoff J, Berrien-Elliott M, et al. Blood natural killer cell deficiency reveals an immunotherapy strategy for atopic dermatitis. Sci Transl Med 2020; 12:12.

26. Schneider L, Tilles S, Lio P, et al. Atopic dermatitis: a practice parameter update 2012. J Allergy Clin Immunol 2013;131(2):295–9, e1-27.

27. Santer M, Rumsby K, Ridd MJ, et al. Adding emollient bath additives to standard eczema management for children with eczema: the BATHE RCT. Health Technol Assess 2018;22:1–116.

28. Quirk S, Rainwater E, Shure A, et al. Vitamin D in atopic dermatitis, chronic urticaria and allergic contact dermatitis. Expert Rev Clin Immunol 2016;12(8): 839–47.

29. Kim G, Bae J. Vitamin D and atopic dermatitis: a systematic review and meta-analysis. Nutrition 2016;32(9):913–20.

30. Schnopp C, Holtmann C, Stock S, et al. Topical steroids under wet-wrap dressings in atopic dermatitis – a vehicle-controlled trial. Dermatology 2002;204:56–9.

31. Papp K, Szepietowski J, Kircik L, et al. Efficacy and safety of ruxolitinib cream for the treatment of atopic dermatitis: results from 2 phase 3, randomized, double-blind studies. J Am Acad Dermatol 2021;85(4):863–72.

32. Garritsen F, Brouwer M, Limpens J, et al. Photo(chemo) therapy in the management of atopic dermatitis: an updated systemic review with implications for practice and research. Br J Dermatol 2014;170:501–13.

33. Drucker A, Eyerich K, de Bruin-Weller M, et al. Use of systemic corticosteroids for atopic dermatitis: International Eczema Council consensus statement. Br J Dermatol 2018;178(3):768–75.

34. Simpson E, Bieber T, Guttman-Yassky E, et al. Two phase 3 trials of dupilumab versus placebo in atopic dermatitis. N Engl J Med 2016;375:2335–48.

35. Blauvelt A, de Bruin-Weller M, Gooderham M, et al. Long-term management of moderate-to-severe atopic dermatitis with dupilumab and concomitant topical corticosteroids (LIBERTY AD CHRONOS): a 1-year, randomized, double-blinded, placebo-controlled, phase 3 trial. Lancet 2017;389:2287–303.

36. Akinlade B, Guttman-Yassky E, de Bruin-Weller M, et al. Conjunctivitis in dupilumab clinical trials. Br J Dermatol 2019;181:459–73.

37. Adbry™ (tralokinumab-ldrm) Prescribing Information. LEO Pharma; December 2021. Available at: https://www.leo-pharma.us/Files/Billeder/US%20Website%20Product%20PIs/AdbryPI.pdf. Accessed March 21, 2022.

38. Worm M, Francuzik W, Kraft M, et al. Modern therapies in atopic dermatitis: biologics and small molecule drugs. Journal Der Deutschen Dermatologischen Gesellschaft 2020;18(10):1085–92.
39. Simpson E, Sinclair R, Forman S, et al. Efficacy and safety of abrocitinib in adults and adolescents with moderate to severe atopic dermatitis (JADE MONO-1): a multicentre, double-blind, randomized, placebo-controlled, phase 3 clinical trial. Lancet 2020;396:255–66.
40. RINVOQ® (upadacitinib) [Package Insert]. North Chicago, Ill.: AbbVie Inc. Available at: https://www.rxabbvie.com/pdf/rinvoq_pi.pdf. Accessed March 21, 2022.
41. Guttman-Yassky E, Thaci D, Pnagan A, et al. Upadacitinib in adults with moderate to severe atopic dermatitis: 16-week results from a randomized, placebo-controlled trial. J Allergy Clin Immunol 2020;145:877–84.

Looks Can Be Deceiving
The Masqueraders of Atopic Dermatitis

Keri Holyoak, MPH, MSHS, PA-C

KEYWORDS

- Atopic dermatitis • Dermatitis • Eczema • Differential diagnosis

KEY POINTS

- AD is a common inflammatory condition seen in all ages and ethnicities with a broad clinical spectrum, differing morphologies, and atypical clinical features.
- Diagnosing AD can be complex because many other skin diseases can potentially mimic AD.
- Balanced consideration of other skin conditions that can resemble, coexist or complicate AD can improve AD management.

INTRODUCTION

AD is a challenging, complex disease for patients and dermatology providers. For the patient, the disease is unpredictable and burdensome with cycles of pruritis, the most burdensome symptom of AD.[1–3] Ill-defined erythematous papules, plaques, excoriations, and serous exudate characterize acute lesions. Extensive scratching of chronic lesions result in thickened, lichenified, hyperpigmented plaques and fibrotic papules. Severity is determined by the extent of erythema, degree of excoriation, and lichenification, intensity of itching and impact on sleep and daily activities.[4] Extreme itching and scratching can lead to irritability, decreased school or work performance, sleep disturbance and issues in interpersonal relationships. These factors can ultimately contribute to neglect and exacerbation of the condition and a negative approach to life.

For dermatology providers, there are a number of masqueraders of AD making it difficult to diagnose. The heterogeneous clinical course of AD and its differing signs, symptoms, and response to treatment can pose a quandary. Without definitive tests to confirm the diagnosis it can be challenging and based heavily on medical history and physical examination. In addition, since the disease can be slow to respond to treatments adherence is another challenge. Despite this high degree of heterogeneity, it is important to recognize AD and be familiar with other skin diseases that can

The Dermatology Center of Salt Lake, 7396 South Union Park Avenue, Suite 201, Midvale, UT 84047, USA
E-mail address: kholyoak@gmail.com

Physician Assist Clin 8 (2023) 717–727
https://doi.org/10.1016/j.cpha.2023.05.007
2405-7991/23/© 2023 Elsevier Inc. All rights reserved.

potentially mimic AD. Those that will be discussed include chronic inflammatory skin conditions, infections, malignancies, and autoimmune conditions.

SEBORRHEIC DERMATITIS

Seborrheic dermatitis (SD) is a very common, chronic condition that causes erythema, scale, and crusting in regions where sebaceous glands are most active. It notably peaks in the first few weeks of life, between 2 weeks and 12 months of age, during adolescence, and adulthood between age 30 and 60 years.[5] It commonly occurs in areas such as the scalp, face (glabella, eyebrows, nasolabial folds, above the upper lip), ears, retro-auricular areas, the upper chest, and body folds (axilla, umbilicus, sub-mammary skin folds, inguinal areas) (**Fig. 1**).[5] A defective epidermal barrier, a hyper-sensitivity to yeast, most commonly *Malassezia*, and sebaceous gland stimulation have been suggested as to the pathogenesis.[6]

Infants often present with greasy, yellow scale with background erythema on the scalp commonly referred to as "cradle cap." Some infants may develop a more diffuse eruption on the trunk and extremities, usually consisting of salmon-pink fine papules coalescing into poorly defined plaques with variable greasy scaling.

Rarely, infants with seborrheic dermatitis develop extensive involvement with eryth-roderma and scaling. Some patients, especially those with more fulminant presenta-tions, may be difficult to distinguish from AD. However, they may also exist on a continuum, with the resolution of seborrheic dermatitis as clinical features of AD be-comes more prominent. In a retrospective review by Alexopoulos and colleagues, the prevalence of AD in patients with infantile seborrheic dermatitis was significantly higher than the rate reported in the general population.[7]

Adolescent or adult seborrheic dermatitis, otherwise known as "dandruff," can pre-sent with fine, flaky scale and mild erythema. It can also present as yellow to orange crusts, greasy scale with erythematous skin on the scalp and central face, retroauric-ular folds, and the upper chest. It is more common in immunocompromised patients and those with neurologic diseases, such as Parkinson's Disease.[8] It can be associ-ated with pruritis, however it is less pruritic than AD (often, there is an absence of pru-ritis) and responds quickly to therapy. Sometimes, symptoms for SD and psoriasis are present, and this condition is referred to as sebopsoriasis underscoring that the clas-sical SD phenotype may just represent one segment in a continuous spectrum of closely related dermatoses.[9,10]

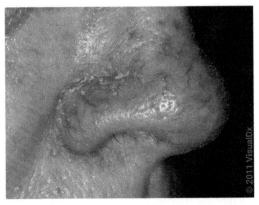

Fig. 1. Scaly, erythematous plaques in the nasolabial folds.

ALLERGIC CONTACT DERMATITIS

Allergic contact dermatitis (ACD) is an inflammatory skin condition caused by a delayed type IV hypersensitivity reaction in response to an allergen or exogenous agent. ACD is often restricted to the areas of the skin that are exposed to the allergen. Severe pruritis, well-demarcated erythematous plaques with edema extending beyond the area of exposure, with overlying vesiculation characterize the acute phase. In subacute phases, scaly or crusty lesions and erosions can develop. The chronic phase features include xerotic crust, lichenification, scaling, and fissuring.

ACD presents after contact with an allergen within 8 to 120 hours in sensitized patients or 12 to 21 days in unsensitized patients.[11] Certain allergens have been found to have higher rates of sensitization among patients with AD when compared with non-atopic patients, including formaldehyde releasers, metal allergens, cocamidopropyl betaine (a surfactant) and fragrances.[12,13] The face (lips, eyelids), neck, forearms, and hands are the most commonly affected areas, followed by the trunk and groin (**Fig. 2**).[14] Metals, preservatives, fragrances, and topical antibiotics are the most frequent causes of allergic contact dermatitis.[15] P-phenylenediamine, commonly used in hair dyes, is also a common sensitizer.[16] Parabens is the most common preservative in cosmetics and pharmaceuticals, but is the least frequent cause of ACD.[17,18]

A skin biopsy is not useful to distinguish ACD from AD, as they share identical histopathologic features. The gold standard for the diagnosis of ACD is patch testing. There are several methods for patch testing, including prepackaged allergen panels, such as the thin-layer rapid use epicutaneous patch test (TRUE test), or customized trays usually performed at a tertiary referral center. Patch test results should be interpreted with clinical context because not all positive results are clinically relevant. This is particularly important in children because allergen panels are developed based on commonly reported allergens in adults; however, children are exposed to a different array of products and thus a close review of their products and environment before patch testing is crucial to increase the diagnostic yield.[19]

The localization of dermatitis to a specific skin area, history of exposure to irritants or potential sensitizers, and relevant patch test positivity suggest the diagnosis of contact dermatitis instead of AD.

PSORIASIS

Psoriasis is a common, chronic, inflammatory, immune-mediated disease affecting 2% to 3% of the general population.[20] A bimodal age distribution is commonly

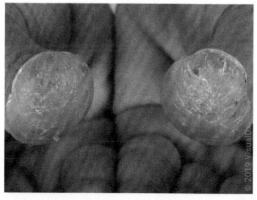

Fig. 2. Scaly plaques with erosion on the distal thumbs.

observed, with the first peak around 20 to 30 years of age and a second peak at 50 to 60 years of age.[21] However, psoriasis can present at any age, from infancy to late adulthood. In contrast to AD, which is typically a T helper (Th)-2 predominant condition, Th1 and Th17 characterize psoriasis. Increased levels of interferon gamma, interleukin (IL)-2, IL-17, IL-22, and IL-23 lead to a robust dermal inflammatory response and proliferation of keratinocytes.[22]

In both pediatric and adult psoriasis, a spectrum of clinical variants exist, including guttate psoriasis, plaque psoriasis, erythrodermic psoriasis, pustular psoriasis, and inverse psoriasis. Plaque psoriasis is the most common clinical subtype and presents with well-demarcated, erythematous plaques with adherent silvery scale commonly located over extensor surfaces.[23] Besides the knees and elbows, psoriasis has a predilection for the scalp, retroauricular creases, gluteal cleft, lower back, and periumbilical area (**Fig. 3**). Occasionally, psoriasis affects the seborrheic areas of the face and scalp, closely mimicking seborrheic dermatitis, as previously mentioned a condition termed sebopsoriasis. Nail findings can be a helpful clue to the diagnosis of psoriasis and include oil spots, irregular pitting, salmon patches, nail thickening, yellowing, and distal onycholysis.[24]

Inverse psoriasis involves the axilla, neck folds, inguinal folds, groin and external genitalia, intergluteal cleft, and umbilicus. Skin lesions of inverse psoriasis tend to display a bright pink-red color and well-defined borders with erythematous smooth plaques that lack scale due to moisture. They appear shiny because of the soft and moist flexural environment. Maceration and superficial erosions are common because sweating and friction can cause irritation and soreness.[25]

Guttate psoriasis occurs more frequently in children than adults and usually presents with an acute onset widespread eruption of small, pink, scaly papules, and plaques.[26] Infectious triggers, particularly streptococcal pharyngitis, have been reported in up to two-thirds of patients with acute onset guttate psoriasis.[27] A history of a preceding respiratory tract infection or sore throat 1 to 2 weeks before an outbreak can help support the diagnosis.[24]

In contrast to AD, the diaper eruption of psoriasis in infants is distinct in appearance, presenting as a large well-demarcated bright red plaque or patch with little scale affecting the buttock and inguinal folds. Commonly referred to as napkin dermatitis, this is the most common presentation of psoriasis in the infant.[28] Psoriasis should be considered in patients with recalcitrant diaper dermatitis.

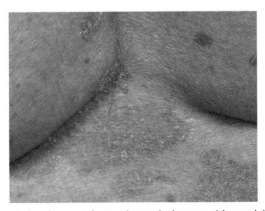

Fig. 3. Well-demarcated, salmon-pink papules and plaques with overlying white scale on the chest and abdomen.

Although the skin is the primary site of involvement, psoriasis is a systemic inflammatory disease process that also commonly affects the joints and the vasculature. The reported prevalence of psoriatic arthritis among patients with psoriasis ranges from 7% to 84%; however, more recent studies estimate that 20% to 30% of patients with psoriasis have psoriatic arthritis.[29,30] Psoriasis has also been associated with an increased risk of metabolic syndrome, cardiovascular events, malignancy, particularly lymphoma, and a decrease in life expectancy.[31]

Although classic psoriasis is usually a clinical diagnosis, the diagnosis can be challenging for infants and young children. A skin biopsy can be performed to confirm the diagnosis and differentiate it from AD. Histologic examination shows regular acanthosis, parakeratosis, thinning of the suprapapillary plate, capillary dilatation, a mononuclear cellular infiltrate, and collections of neutrophils in the epidermis.[32]

SCABIES

Scabies is a common, highly contagious, parasitic skin infection caused by an obligate human parasite, *Sarcoptes scabiei*. Transmission of scabies happens through skin-to-skin contact and indirectly through fomites. It is more often observed in crowded, impoverished living conditions, in elderly nursing home facilities, prisons, and hospitals.[33]

Infestation with *Sarcoptes scabiei* gives the skin an intense pruritus, which, along with few to many erythematous papular lesions, may lead to a mistaken diagnosis of AD. Diagnosis can be made by the visualization of a burrow or linear erythematous scaly track or isolation of a scabies mite often found in burrows in interdigital web spaces, axilla, flexural surfaces of the wrists, belt line, periumbilical skin, genital area, buttocks, periareolar areas in women and the penile shaft in men. In infants and young children, the palms, soles, face, neck, and scalp are frequently involved. However, the lesions caused by scabies are often found in the genital area of adults and the soles of the feet in infants. Secondary skin changes due to severe pruritus are common, including excoriations, eczematization, and crusts, which can mimic AD.[34] Patients with AD develop scabies infections more easily and more severely than other individuals, due to the defect in their skin barrier function.

DERMATOPHYTE INFECTION

Dermatophytosis or tinea is a superficial infection of the hair, skin, and nails caused by dermatophytes, a large group of related fungi. *Trichophyton rubrum* is the most common cause of tinea corporis worldwide.[35]

Tinea corporis, also known as "ringworm," involves the neck, arms, legs, and trunk. It classically presents as an erythematous, annular, or oval, scaly patch with a slightly raised active border and central clearing. Borders of the plaque advance centrifugally and have scale. Multiple plaques can coalesce to form a polycyclic configuration. It is not uncommon for patients to display subtle morphology, resulting in misdiagnosis as AD, nummular eczema, or pityriasis rosea. Partial treatment with topical corticosteroids, known as tinea incognito, commonly leads to alteration in these clinical features and increases the likelihood of misdiagnosis.[36] If suspected, tinea corporis should be ruled out before starting topical corticosteroids.

Tinea manuum involves one or both hands and frequently occurs with tinea pedis.[37] It presents as erythematous, scaly and dry, hyperkeratotic palms and is frequently confused with AD, ACD, or palmar psoriasis.

Tinea capitis, a dermatophyte infection of the scalp, is commonly seen in children, particularly of African American descent, and rarely seen in adults. Findings can range from subtle with a fine noninflammatory scale, which can be mistaken for seborrheic dermatitis or AD, to inflammatory boggy alopecic scaly plaques. The presence of diffuse or patchy alopecia, pustules, broken hairs, or posterior auricular lymphade-nopathy warrants a work-up for tinea capitis before considering alternative diagnoses.

Potassium-hydroxide (KOH) wet-mount preparations can be painlessly performed in the office to confirm the diagnosis with the presence of branching hyphae, pseudo-hyphae, or budding yeast. Scraping of the scale can also be sent for fungal culture. Alternatively, a skin biopsy can be performed with a Periodic acid-Schiff (PAS) stain, which will highlight the presence of fungal elements in the stratum corneum.

CUTANEOUS T-CELL LYMPHOMA

Patients with cutaneous T-cell lymphomas (CTCL) may have an eczematous appearance in the early stages, with numerous variants and clinical appearances, and is often misdiagnosed as AD. Mycosis fungoides (MF) and Sezary syndrome (SS) are the most common forms of CTCL, compromising more than half of the cases with an overall incidence of MF/SS of approximately 4 per 1 million people.[38] Rarely seen in childhood and adolescence, MF typically affects adults with a median age of 55 to 60 year old. Up to one-third of patients with MF report AD as a prior diagnosis.[39]

In classic MF, 3 clinical morphologies (patch, plaque, and tumor) are recognized. Early disease presents as well-defined, scaly, erythematous patches or thin plaques with atrophic surfaces in non-sun-exposed areas, the so-called "bathing suit" distribution, such as the chest, breasts, lower trunk, thighs, buttocks, and groin.[40] Early-stage MF is indolent and a very slowly progressive disease that can evolve over many years to decades to more widespread and advanced stages characterized by infiltrative plaques, cutaneous tumors, erythroderma, and eventually nodal and visceral involvement (**Fig. 4**).

Hypopigmented MF more commonly affects the pediatric population especially those with darker skin types, Fitzpatrick skin types III-VI.[40] It is characterized by round, oval, or irregular nonatrophic hypopigmented macules and patches with fine scaling. Hypopigmented lesions of MF frequently resemble pityriasis alba and are usually asymptomatic with little to no pruritis; however, the involvement of the "bathing suit" distribution, and fine scale can help distinguish hypopigmented MF.

A skin biopsy is required to confirm the diagnosis of MF and will demonstrate a dermal infiltrate composed of lymphocytes with hyperchromatic and irregularly

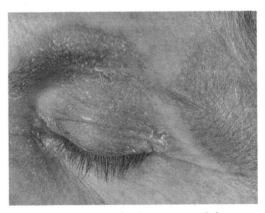

Fig. 4. Well-demarcated, erythematous scaly plaques around the eye.

contoured nuclei with epidermotropism.[39] These findings are often subtle and serial biopsies may be required if there is a high index of suspicion.

Immunohistochemical studies showing a CD4+ predominant infiltrate with loss of CD7+ staining can help verify the diagnosis of MF. The infiltrate in hypopigmented MF may be composed predominantly of CD8+ T cells rather than CD4+ T cells.[39] T-cell rearrangement studies are performed on tissue to confirm clonality.

Lymph nodes, peripheral blood, and/or visceral organs may be clinically involved. All patients warrant a complete physical examination with palpation for lymph nodes, complete blood count with differential, comprehensive metabolic panel, and lactate dehydrogenase. Tumor stage of the disease is considered the most important predictor of disease-specific survival.[41]

PITYRIASIS LICHENOIDES CHRONICA

Pityriasis lichenoides chronica (PLC) is an idiopathic, generally benign, T-cell lymphoproliferative disorder that exists on a clinical spectrum with pityriasis lichenoides et varioliformis acuta (PLEVA), the more acute form, and febrile ulceronecrotic Mucha-Habermann disease (FUMHD), which is more severe, generalized, and associated with systemic symptoms.[42] The incidence of PLC is estimated at 1 in 2000 people, and 20% of these cases affecting children, with the peak incidence between 5 and 10 years of age.[43]

The development of PLC is usually gradual and characterized by the development of numerous red-brown papules on the trunk, buttocks, and proximal extremities. The eruption is usually asymptomatic, however, associated pruritis occurs in some patients. Lesions can relapse and regress over months to years, leaving behind hypopigmentated and hyperpigmentated macules or patches with no scarring (**Fig. 5**). In a retrospective study of 46 children with PCL, the median duration of disease was 20 months (range 3–132 months).[43]

In most cases, PLC is a benign, self-limited, condition that may last for years but usually spontaneously resolves. However, there are reports, more commonly in adults, of PLC in association with cutaneous T-cell lymphoma, thus requiring regular clinical monitoring in these patients.[44]

DERMATOMYOSITIS

Dermatomyositis (DM) is a chronic, complex immune-mediated condition mainly affecting the skin and skeletal muscle. It is seen in adults at an estimated rate of 5 to

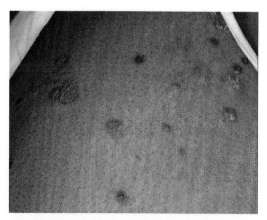

Fig. 5. Numerous, scaly, flat-topped, pink, and violaceous papules.

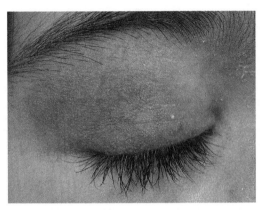

Fig. 6. Eyelid erythema of heliotrope rash.

11 cases per 100,000 per year, and children at an estimated rate of 2 to 3 children per million per year.[45,46] It has a bimodal age distribution, with 2 peaks occurring between 4 and 14 years of age (juvenile DM) and between 40 and 60 years of age (adult DM).[47]

Classic DM is characterized by an inflammatory myopathy with associated cutaneous findings, which frequently precede muscle involvement and thus represent an opportunity for early diagnosis.[45]

The most common and pathognomoic skin lesions are violaceous to erythematous flat-topped papules with fine scale overlying the elbows and knees (Gottron sign) and distal and proximal interphalangeal joints (Gottron papules). Early in the disease course, these lesions are often mistaken for AD due to their extensor distribution and morphology composed of scaly erythematous papules.

Symmetric periorbital violaceous erythema that is more pronounced over the upper eyelids, or the heliotrope rash, is another feature of DM (**Fig. 6**). Nail bed changes, including ragged cuticles and periungual telangiectasias, can serve as other clinical clues to the diagnosis of DM. Additional diagnostic clinical features include poikilodermatous change commonly over the upper chest and shoulders (Shawl sign) and lateral thighs (Holster sign). In darker skin types in particular, poikilodermatous change can be mistaken for erythema associated with AD.

The presence of the pathognomonic cutaneous findings with 2 to 3 clinical signs of myositis (progressive symmetric proximal muscle weakness, muscle biopsy with evidence of myositis, elevation of muscle-derived serum enzyme levels, and/or evidence of myopathy on MRI) secures the diagnosis.[48]

SUMMARY

AD is a common inflammatory condition seen in all ages and ethnicities with a broad clinical spectrum and atypical clinical features. Knowledge of AD's constellation of features and differential diagnosis is important for all those that care for patients. Balanced consideration of these aspects can improve AD diagnosis and management.

CLINICS CARE POINTS

- Without definitive tests to confirm the diagnosis of AD it can be challenging and based heavily on medical history and physical examination.

- It is important to recognize AD and be familiar with other skin diseases that can potentially mimic AD.
- Common differential diagnoses for atopic dermatitis include seborrheic dermatitis, allergic contact dermatitis, dermatophyte infection, psoriasis, scabies, cutaneous T-cell lymphoma, pityriasis lichenoides chronica, and dermatomyositis.

DISCLOSURE

The author has no relevant financial interests to declare.

REFERENCES

1. Laughter M, Maymome M, Mashayekhi S, et al. The Global Burden of Disease of Atopic Dermatitis from 1990–2017. Br J Dermatol 2021;184(2):E42.
2. Kim J, Chao L, Simpson E, et al. Persistence of atopic dermatitis (AD): a systemic review and meta-analysis. J Am Acad Dermatol 2016;75(4):681–7.
3. Eichenfield L, Wynnis T, Chamlin S, et al. Guidelines of care for the management of atopic dermatitis: section 1. Diagnosis and assessment of atopic dermatitis. J Am Acad Dermatol 2014;70(2):338–51.
4. Lio P, Lee M, LeBovidge J, et al. Clinical management of atopic dermatitis: practical highlights and updates from the Atopic Dermatitis Practice Parameter 2012. J Allergy Clin Immunol Pract 2014;2(4):361–9.
5. Suh D. Seborrheic Dermatitis. In: Kang S, Amagai M, Bruckner A, et al, editors. Fitzpatrick's dermatology. 9th ed. United States: McGraw Hill; 2019. p. 428.
6. Borda L, Wikramanayake T. Seborrheic dermatitis and dandruff: a comprehensive review. J Clin Investig Dermatol 2015;3:1–22.
7. Alexopoulos A, Kakourou T, Orfanou I, et al. Retrospective analysis of the relationship between infantile seborrheic dermatitis and atopic dermatitis. Pediatr Dermatol 2014;31:125–30.
8. Dessinioti C, Katsambas A. Seborrheic Dermatitis: etiology, risk factors, and treatments: facts and controversies. Clin Dermatol 2013;31:343.
9. Tull T, Noy M, Bunker C, et al. Sebopsoriasis in patients with HIV: a case series of 20 patients. Br J Dermatol 2017;176:813.
10. Wikramanayake T, Borda L, Miteva M, et al. Seborrheic dermatitis- Looking beyond Malassezia. Exp Dermatol 2019;991–1001.
11. Chan C, Zug K. Diagnosis and Management of Dermatitis, Including Atopic, Contact and Hand Eczemas. Med Clin 2021;105(4):611–26.
12. Shaughnessy C, Malajian D, Belsito D. Cutaneous delayed-type hypersensitivity in patients with atopic dermatitis: reactivity to topical preservatives. J Am Acad Dermatol 2014;70:102–7.
13. Malajian D, Belsito D. Cutaneous delayed-type hypersensitivity in patients with atopic dermatitis. J Am Acad Dermatol 2013;69:232–7.
14. Shaughnessy C, Malajian D, Belsito D. Cutaneous delayed-type hypersensitivity in patients with atopic dermatitis: reactivity to surfactants. J Am Acad Dermatol 2014;70:704–8.
15. Herro E, Matiz C, Sullivan K, et al. Frequency of contact allergens in pediatric patients with atopic dermatitis. J Clin Aesthet Dermatol 2011;4:39–41.
16. Militello G, Jacob S, Crawford G. Allergic contact dermatitis in children. Curr Opin Pediatr 2006;18:385–90.
17. Sasseville D. Hypersensitivity to preservatives. Dermatol Ther 2004;17(3):251.

18. Zug K, Warshaw E, Fowler J, et al. Patch-test results of the North American Contact Dermatitis Group 2005-2006. Marks J Dermatitis 2009;20(3):149.

19. de Waard-van der Spek F, Darsow U, Mortz C, et al. EAACI position paper for practical patch testing in allergic contact dermatitis in children. Pediatr Allergy Immunol 2015;26:598–606.

20. Michalek I, Loring B, John S. A systematic review of worldwide epidermiology of psoriasis. J Eur Acad Dermatol Veneroel 2017;31(2):205–12.

21. Rachakond T, Schupp C, Armstrong A. Psoriasis prevalence among adults in the United States. J Am Acad Dermatol 2017;76(3):377–90.

22. Shah K. Diagnosis and treatment of pediatric psoriasis: current and future. Am J Clin Dermatol 2013;14:195–213.

23. Morris A, Rogers M, Fischer G, et al. Childhood psoriasis: a clinical review of 1262 cases. Pediatr Dermatol 2001;18:188–98.

24. Leman J, Burden D. Psoriasis in children: a guide to its diagnosis and management. Paediatr Drugs 2001;3:673–80.

25. Merola J, Qureshi A, Husni M. Underdiagnosed and undertreated psoriasis: nuances of treating psoriasis affecting the scalp, face, intertriginous areas, genitals, hands, feet, and nails. Dermatol Ther 2018;31(3):e12589.

26. Verbov J. Psoriasis in childhood. Arch Dis Child 1992;67:75–6.

27. Fry L, Baker B. Triggering psoriasis: the role of infections and medications. Clin Dermatol 2007;25:606–15.

28. Burden-Teh E, Thomas K, Ratib S, et al. The epidemiology of childhood psoriasis: a scoping review. Br J Dermatol 2016;174:1242–57.

29. López Estebaránz J, Zarco-Montejo P, Samaniego M, et al. Prevalence and clinical features of psoriatic arthritis in psoriasis patients in Spain. Limitations of PASE as a screening tool. Eur J Dermatol 2015;25:57–63.

30. Pedersen O, Svendsen A, Ejstrup L, et al. The occurrence of psoriatic arthritis in Denmark. Ann Rheum Dis 2008;67:1422–6.

31. Johnson M, Armstrong A. Clinical and histologic diagnostic guidelines for psoriasis: a critical review. Clin Rev Allergy Immunol 2013;44:166–72.

32. Balato A, Scalvenzi M, Cirillo T, et al. Psoriasis in children: a review. Curr Pediatr Rev 2015;11:10–26.

33. Hengge U, Currie B, Jäger G, et al. Scabies: a ubiquitous neglected skin disease. Lancet Infect Dis 2006;6:769–79.

34. Heukelbach J, Feldmeier H. Scabies. Lancet 2006;367:1767–74.

35. Kelly B. Superficial fungal infections. Pediatr Rev 2012;33:e22–37.

36. Alston S, Cohen B, Braun M. Persistent and recurrent tinea corporis in children treated with combination antifungal/corticosteroid agents. Pediatrics 2003;111: 201–3.

37. Baumgardner D. Fungal infections from human and animal contact. J Pateint cent Res Rev 2017;4(2):78–89.

38. Foss FM, Girardi M. Mycosis fungoides and sezary syndrome. Hematol Oncol Clin North Am 2017;31(2):297–315.

39. Boulos S, Vaid R, Aladily T, et al. Clinical presentation, immunopathology, and treatment of juvenile-onset mycosis fungoides: a case series of 34 patients. J Am Acad Dermatol 2014;71:1117–26.

40. Onsun N, Kural Y, Su O, et al. Hypopigmented mycosis fungoides associated with atopy in two children. Pediatr Dermatol 2006;23:493–6.

41. Agar N, Wedgeworth E, Crichton S, et al. Survival outcomes and prognostic factors in mycosis fungoides/Sézary syndrome: validation of the revised

International Society for Cutaneous Lymphomas/European Organisation for Research and Treatment of Cancer staging proposal. J Clin Oncol 2010;28: 4730–9.

42. Bowers S, Warshaw E. Pityriasis lichenoides and its subtypes. J Am Acad Dermatol 2006;55:557–72.

43. Brazzelli V, Carugno R, Rivetti N, et al. Narrowband UVB phototherapy for pediatric generalized pityriasis lichenoides. Photodermatol Photoimmunol Photomed 2013;29:330–3.

44. Ersoy-Evans S, Greco M, Mancini A. Pityriasis lichenoides in childhood: a retrospective review of 124 patients. J Am Acad Dermatol 2007;56(2):205–10.

45. Iaccarino L, Ghirardello A, Bettio S, et al. The clinical features, diagnosis and classification of dermatomyositis. J Autoimmun 2014;48-49:122–7.

46. Almeida B, Campanilho-Marques R, Arnold K, et al. Analysis of published criteria for clinically inactive disease in a large juvenile dermatomyositis cohort shows that skin disease is underestimated. Arthritis Rheumatol 2015;67:2495–502.

47. Dewane M, Waldman R, Lu J. Dermatomyositis; clinical features and pathogenesis. J Am Acad Dermatol 2020;82(2):267–81.

48. Barrett M, Minnelly L. Differential Diagnosis of Atopic Dermatitis. Immunol Allergy Clin 2017;37(1):11–34.

Anaphylaxis
What You Need to Know

Nicole Soucy, MPAS, PA-C[a],*, Amanda Michaud, DMSc, PA-C, AE-C[b]

KEYWORDS

• Anaphylaxis • Allergy • Venom • Latex • Drug • Food

KEY POINTS

• Anaphylaxis is a life-threatening emergency that can be caused by various mechanisms.
• Prompt treatment of anaphylaxis with epinephrine is necessary for the best outcomes.
• Patients should be educated on their condition and provided emergency plans and on-demand treatment.

INTRODUCTION

Anaphylaxis is a severe, acute, life-threatening systemic allergic reaction that can result in various possible presentations.[1,2] The most common causes of anaphylaxis are foods, drugs, stinging insects, and latex. In adults, the most common causes of anaphylaxis are medications and stinging insects. In children, the most common trigger is food. The overall prevalence of anaphylaxis is estimated to occur between 1.6% to 5.1% of the United States population.[1] Death from anaphylaxis is rare due to increased recognition of the condition and treatment modalities. First-line therapy includes intramuscular epinephrine, but this potentially life-saving medication is often underutilized.

DEFINITION

There has been discourse regarding the exact definition of anaphylaxis due to the evolution of our understanding of the potential mechanisms involved and various clinical presentations. The lack of a universal consensus among the allergy, asthma, immunology community has resulted in professional organizations outlining different definitions. In short, the current definition of anaphylaxis from the American Academy of Allergy, Asthma and Immunology (AAAAI) and the American College of Allergy, Asthma, and Immunology (ACAAI) is "an acute, life-threatening systemic reaction

[a] UT Southwestern, Association of Physician Assistants in Allergy, Asthma, and Immunology, Board of Directors; [b] Allergy & Immunology Family Allergy and Asthma Consultants, Association of Physician Assistants in Allergy, Asthma, and Immunology, Board of Directors
* Corresponding author. 2350 North Stemmons Freeway F6601.01, Dallas, TX 75207.
E-mail address: nicolesoucypac@gmail.com

Physician Assist Clin 8 (2023) 729–738
https://doi.org/10.1016/j.cpha.2023.05.008
2405-7991/23/© 2023 Elsevier Inc. All rights reserved.
physicianassistant.theclinics.com

with varied mechanisms, clinical presentations, and severity that results from the sudden release of mediators from mast cells and basophils."[1,2]

PATHOPHYSIOLOGY

The pathophysiology of anaphylaxis usually involves the binding of IgE molecules to the IgE receptor present on the surface of mast cells and basophils. This binding causes these cells to degranulate and release molecules that promote vasodilation and inflammation. However, there are other mechanisms involved in some types of anaphylaxis that may include cytokines (such as IL-6 or IL-10) or complement components. Other possible cell types involved in anaphylaxis include neutrophils, monocytes, macrophages, and other signaling molecules. It is important to recognize that while the most common pathway that leads to anaphylaxis is an IgE-mediated pathway, there are other potential pathways involved.[1] Regardless of the pathway taken, the end result is the release of mediators that promote vasodilation and inflammation which results in substantial systemic symptoms.

SIGNS/SYMPTOMS

Anaphylaxis can have variable presentations. The mechanism of action of anaphylaxis (most commonly, the release of mediators from mast cells and basophils) can affect multiple organ systems, particularly in the skin, pulmonary, cardiac, and gastrointestinal tissue. Up to 90% of patients will experience cutaneous symptoms such as urticaria, angioedema, flushing, and pruritus.[3] The presence of cutaneous symptoms in a patient suspected to be experiencing anaphylaxis can be a useful–but not foolproof–diagnostic aid. Multiple organ systems can be involved simultaneously. Half of the patients will experience respiratory symptoms and approximately one-third of patients will experience cardiac symptoms. Rarely, atypical symptoms such as headache, substernal chest pain, or seizure can occur during anaphylaxis. Potential variations in the presentation of anaphylaxis can make diagnosis difficult (**Fig. 1**).

DIAGNOSIS

Clinicians currently lack diagnostic tools that are sensitive and specific enough to definitvely identify anaphylaxis, which can make diagnosis difficult. The current laboratory tests available to evaluate acute anaphylaxis are limited and can be falsely negative even in the face of true anaphylaxis.[1] Given that anaphylaxis is a rapid, life-threatening condition, waiting for laboratory evaluation for confirmation can hinder the evaluation and treatment in the emergent setting.

The National Institute of Allergy and Infectious Disease (NIAID) and the Food Allergy and Anaphylaxis Network (FAAN) released guidelines in 2006 with the intent to help facilitate the rapid diagnosis of anaphylaxis in the emergency care setting. These guidelines have demonstrated 95% sensitivity and about 71% specificity in recognizing anaphylaxis.[1,4] Three different "scenarios" of anaphylaxis fall within this criterion, as shown in **Table 1**.[4] All scenarios require a sudden onset of symptoms. There are variations in the criteria depending on suspicion of allergen consumption and body systems affected (**Table 1**).

LABORATORY EVALUATION

Laboratory evaluation is not usually completed during acute anaphylaxis, in favor of a focus on stabilizing the patient.[1] However, if laboratory events are obtained during an event of suspected anaphylaxis, serum tryptase is shown to be the most useful.[3]

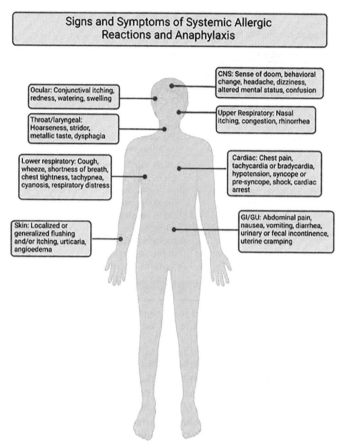

Fig. 1. Signs and symptoms of systemic allergic reactions and anaphylaxis. (Created with biorender.com.)

Plasma histamine levels, 24-hour urinary histamine metabolites, and urinary prostaglandin D2 may also be ordered to aid in the diagnosis, but are not routinely utilized.

Other laboratory studies may be ordered to evaluate for other conditions that may mimic anaphylaxis. Outside of the acute anaphylactic event, further evaluation can be done in the allergy specialty setting to confirm the etiology of anaphylaxis. This workup may include a baseline serum tryptase as well as evaluation for IgE-mediated allergy through skin prick testing or specific IgE serum testing. This evaluation sometimes includes testing for uncommon causes of anaphylaxis, such as complement deficiencies or sensitivity to galactose-1,3,-α-galactose. It is important to know that the overall specificity of allergy skin prick or serum IgE testing remains poor, and large panel-specific IgE serum testing is not recommended. Testing should be limited to potential triggers of concern.[5]

CAUSES OF ANAPHYLAXIS
Food allergy

Foods are the most common cause of anaphylaxis, especially in children.[3] While any food protein could cause an allergic reaction, the most common foods known to cause anaphylaxis are peanuts, tree nuts, fish, shellfish, milk, and egg. The incidence of

Table 1
NIAID/FAAN diagnostic criteria for anaphylaxis[4]

	Scenario 1	Scenario 2	Scenario 3
Primary criteria	Sudden onset of illness *with the involvement of the skin and mucosal tissue*	Sudden onset of illness	Sudden reduced blood pressure[a]
Allergen consumption	Regardless of allergen consumption	Likely exposure to an allergen	Confirmed exposure to a known allergen
Secondary criteria	At least *ONE* of the following Sudden respiratory symptoms Sudden reduced blood pressure Symptoms of end organ dysfunction	At least *TWO* of the following Skin or mucosal involvement Sudden respiratory symptoms A sudden decrease in blood pressure Symptoms of end organ dysfunction Sudden GI symptoms	None

[a] Defined as a > 30% drop in systolic blood pressure for the patient OR Systolic blood pressure <90 mm Hg (adults) or lower than average age defined blood pressure in pediatric patients.

sesame allergy is rising in the United States, and it is now considered a common cause of food allergy.[6] The "top 9" most common food allergens are outlined in **Box 1**. Diagnosis of food-induced allergic reactions should be made after thorough history taking, including information about the timing of the reaction, symptoms experienced, duration, and treatments attempted. Avoidance of the offending food is the mainstay of food allergy management.[3] Immunotherapy for food allergy is an emerging treatment option to raise the threshold of reactivity and help prevent allergic reactions after accidental ingestion.[7]

All patients with food allergy should have access to an epinephrine auto-injector and have an emergency care plan that is updated annually.[3] It is impossible to predict the severity of a future reaction based on past reactions and strict avoidance and

Box 1
Common allergenic foods

Egg

Milk

Soy

Wheat

Peanut

Tree Nut

Shellfish

Fish

Sesame

diligence is necessary for patients and caregivers to adhere to, even if prior reactions were previously mild. Some patients, such as adolescents or those with asthma history, are at increased risk of more severe allergic reactions.

Stinging insect allergy

Most stings from fire ants, bees, hornets, yellow jackets, and wasps—while bothersome—are not life threatening. Most stings from these insects present with pain, swelling, and possibly itching localized to the site of the sting. In those who experience large, localized reactions, the risk of systemic reaction to subsequent stings is estimated to be 5-10%.[8,9] Severe systemic allergic reactions to insect stings affect up to 0.8% of children and 3% of adults in the United States.[8] Up to 60% of patients with a history of systemic reaction to insect stings will experience another systemic allergic reaction on a subsequent sting.[8,9] It is, therefore, strongly recommended that these individuals undergo diagnostic testing for stinging insect allergy and consider the option for venom immunotherapy (VIT).

A thorough history and referral to an allergy subspectialist for skin testing is necessary for the diagnosis of a stinging insect allergy. In some cases, serum-specific IgE testing to insect venoms can be completed in lieu of skin testing. There are commercially available extracts to skin test for honeybee, yellow jacket, white faced hornet, yellow hornet, wasp, and fire ant. Patients with a history of systemic reaction to a stinging insect and positive skin prick testing are eligible for VIT. Patients with venom allergy are at higher risk of having a comorbid mast cell disorder, such as mastocytosis.[8] Evaluation for mastocytosis can be done in the allergy subspeciality setting and often includes a baseline serum tryptase level.

Avoidance of the causative stinging insects is key in patients with venom allergy. Considering virtually all exposures are accidental, patients with venom allergy must be educated on proper avoidance measures and need to carry an epinephrine autoinjector. Some avoidance measures can include avoiding the preparation of or eating food while outdoors, avoiding flowering plants, keeping trash cans covered, and avoidance of treading barefoot when outdoors.[9]

Drug allergy

Medications are the second-most common cause of anaphylaxis.[3,10] The most common classes of medications known to cause anaphylaxis are antibiotics, non-steroidal anti-inflammatory drugs (NSAIDs), monoclonal antibodies, chemotherapeutic agents, and radiocontrast media.[10] In the perioperative setting, common triggers include neuromuscular blocking agents, antibiotics, opioids, latex, and blood-product transfusions.

β-lactam antibiotics are the most common cause of antibiotic-induced anaphylaxis. The most established testing protocols exist for penicillin and β-lactams.[3,10] When penicillin allergy is suspected, patients can undergo standardized skin testing and oral ingestion challenge in the office setting. Unfortunately, skin testing is not available for all drugs due to a lack of established non-irritating concentrations of many drugs. This can lead to difficulty in diagnosis of non-penicillin drug allergies.

Radiocontrast media reactions can also cause anaphylactic events, but may be safe for future administrationwith premedication and using the lowest-molecular weight contrast media.[3] This requires evaluation in the allergy subspeciality office to determine potential risks and benefits, as well as to evaluate for possible alternatives.

Latex allergy

Prevalence of natural rubber latex (NRL) allergy in the general population ranges from 1 to 7.6%.[11] Risk factors for the development of NRL allergy includes occupation, history of more than five surgical procedures, presence of various congenital or neurological disease (such as spina-bifida), and a history of atopy. Common occupations with higher risk of latex exposures include health care, hairdressers, housekeeping, and food handling.

Symptoms of NRL allergy can be variable and can range from mild symptoms—such as contact urticaria—to anaphylaxis. Anaphylaxis to NRL most commonly occurs during surgery and during medical or dental procedures. Perioperative NRL allergic reactions can be severe. It is important to note that NRL also has the potential to induce a non-IgE-mediated type IV allergic contact dermatitis, which results in a delayed-type cutaneous rash without other systemic symptoms. This is not to be confused with an IgE-mediated NRL allergy, which has the potential to be life threatening. Making this distinction is typically done in the allergy subspeciality setting.

There is no standardized reagent for skin prick testing for latex available in the United States, which can make diagnosis challenging. Diagnosis relies on the clinical history and detection of specific IgE to latex. Unfortunately, specific IgE testing to NRL has a sensitivity of only 70-80% and false negatives can be seen.[11] Like food allergy, challenge tests are considered the gold standard for diagnosis, especially if the diagnosis is unclear. After the diagnosis of an IgE-mediated NRL allergy has been made, patients must be educated on the avoidance of latex. Patients should have an epinephrine auto-injector prescribed. Approximately 21-58% of individuals with NRL allergy will also react to certain "latex fruits" such as banana, avocado, kiwi, and chestnut.[11] This condition is known as latex-fruit syndrome and these patients should avoid these fruits along with latex.

Other allergic conditions and co-factors

Other, more uncommon, allergic or immune-mediated conditions that can cause anaphylaxis include exercise-induced anaphylaxis, alpha-gal syndrome, cold-induced urticaria, cholinergic urticaria, idiopathic anaphylaxis, or seminal fluid allergy.[3] Alpha-gal allergy should be suspected if a patient has an anaphylactic reaction several hours after eating mammalian meat. Cold-induced or cholinergic urticaria should be suspected in patients who develop anaphylaxis after exposure to cold or elevated temperatures, respectively. Exercise is an important cause of anaphylaxis and can also be a co-factor contributing to the development and severity of allergic reactions.[3] **Box 2** outlines potential co-factors that can potentiate or increase the risk for an anaphylactic reaction.[3,12]

Box 2
Cofactors that can potentiate the risk of anaphylaxis

Sleep deprivation

Hormonal changes

Infection

Alcohol/drug use

Certain medications

Unstable asthma

Underlying mast cell disease

High pollen levels

Differential diagnosis

A detailed history is paramount in the evaluation of an individual with a suspected history of anaphylaxis. It is also important to consider a comprehensive differential diagnosis, as there are many other syndromes that can mimic anaphylaxis or allergic reactions.[3] The differential diagnosis for anaphylaxis is vast. Conditions commonly mistaken as anaphylaxis include vasovagal reactions, vocal cord disorders, panic attacks, food poisoning, drug-induced flushing, carcinoid syndrome, and pheochromocytoma. This, however, is not an exhaustive list and additional differentials are outlined in **Table 2**.[3] Various elements of the patient's history and laboratory diagnostics can be helpful if the diagnosis is not clear.

MANAGEMENT
Acute treatment

The prompt administration of epinephrine is the first-line treatment for anaphylaxis.[3] If possible, the offending trigger should be removed — such as stopping an intravenous infusion triggering the reaction. The patient should be assessed for a patent airway and adequate circulation. Evaluation for signs of respiratory distress, cardiovascular compromise, and altered mental status is also necessary. If needed, cardiopulmonary resuscitation should commence, and emergency medical services (EMS) notified. Most acute allergic reactions can be managed in the office setting, but EMS transport may be necessary to a higher level of care in cases of severe anaphylaxis or when there is a lack of adequate response to epinephrine.

Patients experiencing anaphylaxis should be placed in the supine position but may need to be placed upright if experiencing significant respiratory symptoms.[12] The left lateral semi-recumbent position is preferred in pregnant patients. Patients should be under direct observation by medical staff members and ongoing status monitored.[3] Epinephrine 1:1000 is given to adults at 0.3 mg dosage and in children from 0.1mg to 0.3 mg dosage depending on weight. Dosing can be repeated after five minutes if symptoms are still present. Commercially available epinephrine auto-injectors come in strengths of 0.1 mg, 0.15 mg, and 0.3 mg per dose. Patients with severe reactions should be monitored in a health care setting for 4-8 hours.

Table 2 Differential diagnosis of anaphylaxis by system	
Cutaneous	Generalized urticaria Hereditary/acquired angioedema Medication-induced angioedema
Pulmonary	Asthma exacerbation Pulmonary embolism Vocal cord dysfunction Hyperventilation syndrome
Cardiac	Cerebrovascular accident Myocardial infarction Capillary leak syndrome
Neurologic	Seizure Syncope
Psychiatric	Anxiety/panic attack
Gastrointestinal	Scombroid fish poisoning Food poisoning

Adjunctive medications include supplemental oxygen as well as nebulized beta-agonists for patients with respiratory symptoms or signs of bronchospasm.[3,12] If a patient is on a beta blocker, the effects of epinephrine may be reduced. In those instances, it may be necessary to administer glucagon. Angiotensin-converting enzyme (ACE) inhibitors have been found to potentially contribute to more severe anaphylaxis. Some allergists discourage their use with allergen immunotherapy or in patients with venom allergy.[3] Patients with cardiovascular compromise should be administered intravenous fluids.[12] Advanced airway management or use of vasopressors may be necessary in the hospital setting, if needed.

It is imperative to note that oral or systemic antihistamines or corticosteroids should never be administered as first-line therapy for patients with suspected anaphylaxis, as these medications are helpful only as supplemental medications. Corticosteroids and antihistamines do not treat anaphylaxis, prevent airway obstruction, or treat hypotension.[12] There is conflicting data and overall lack of strong evidence that corticosteroids can help prevent secondary, or biphasic, allergic reactions from occurring. There is no evidence of the benefit of antihistamines for anaphylaxis, but oral antihistamines may be used for mild allergic reactions (such as localized urticaria). Oral second-generation cetirizine is preferred over diphenhydramine due to faster onset of action and a reduced side effect profile.

Long-term management

Avoidance is key when a trigger to anaphylaxis is known. All patients who have experienced anaphylaxis or are at risk of experiencing anaphylaxis should carry an epinephrine auto-injector. Patients at risk of or who have experienced anaphylaxis should also be referred to an allergist for proper identification, confirmation of the diagnosis, education, and long-term management of their condition.[3,12] Working with an allergist can provide diagnostic expertise when needed to clarify the causative agent or if the offending agent is unclear. In addition to diagnostics, allergists can provide ongoing education and monitoring of the allergy and risk of future allergic reactions. Under the care of an allergy clinician, immunomodulatory treatment options including food immunotherapy, VIT, or medication desensitization may be considered.[12] Some food allergies can be outgrown in childhood, and an allergist can properly guide families and patients on safe introduction, when applicable.

An anaphylaxis or emergency action plan outlining clear steps to be taken should a reaction occur should be created, updated, and reviewed annually in the allergy subspeciality setting. Concurrent risk factors, such as poorly controlled asthma, cardiovascular disease, or risk-taking behavior should also be addressed to minimize the risk of severe anaphylaxis.

DISCUSSION

Our evolving understanding of anaphylaxis has presented with it unique challenges in identifying exactly what anaphylaxis is, resulting in disagreement on a precise definition. This lack of unity has, in some ways, contributed to confusion among clinicians on identification and, in some cases, proper treatment of anaphylaxis. The medical community, as it expands its understanding on the nuances of anaphylaxis, should strive to develop a more universal definition of anaphylaxis to limit confusion.

The most common triggers of anaphylaxis include food, drugs, stinging insects, and latex. Often times, the biggest challenge in treating patients with previous anaphylaxis is identifying the causative trigger. Much like a detective solving a crime, allergy specialists often have to sleuth to come to the correct conclusions. It is for this reason that a careful, detailed history is worth its weight in gold when evaluating a patient who has experienced anaphylaxis. Skin prick testing and specific IgE testing can be performed to help aid diagnosis when the diagnosis is unclear from the history alone. Ultimately, oral challenges, when applicable, are considered to be the gold standard to diagnosis of a food allergy and for some medications. It becomes more challenging, however, when there is limited diagnostic testing available for a particular trigger, as we see with drug allergy.

The overarching theme of anaphylaxis is the need for prompt administration of epinephrine. The NIAID/FAAN guidelines have attempted to streamline the quick identification of symptoms of anaphylaxis and thus aid clinicians in providing quick treatment with epinephrine. Still, there continues to be misconceptions among clinicians and patients alike in the identification and proper treatment of anaphylaxis. Studies show that anaphylaxis is not properly treated with antihistamines and corticosteroids, yet these medications are still frequently utilized by some clinicians as "first-line" treatment, rather than epinephrine.

Laboratory testing is not generally useful in the acute setting of anaphylaxis and is often not utilized. Prompt treatment with epinephrine should be promptly administered in patients experiencing anaphylaxis. If laboratory testing is pursued after treatment, a serum tryptase level may help confirm the diagnosis. However, a negative serum tryptase level does not rule out anaphylaxis.

Proper education and training for patients who are at risk of experiencing an anaphylactic reaction are of paramount importance. Careful outlines of what to do in an emergency are essential for patients at risk of experiencing anaphylaxis and should be thoroughly reviewed with patients. Having a care plan available for patients can help limit confusion and stress the need for prompt use of epinephrine. Training of how to utilize an epinephrine auto-injector can translate into proper administration during an actual emergency. Like periodic fire drills in schools, patients and caregivers should also consider "anaphylaxis" drills so that they are prepared in the event of an emergency.

SUMMARY

Anaphylaxis is an acute, potentially life-threatening systemic allergic reaction with various presentations and triggers. The variable signs and symptoms of anaphylaxis can lead to delayed recognition, and it is important for clinicians to be aware of the numerous presentations. The most common causes of anaphylaxis are due to foods, drugs, venoms, and latex. A careful history and diagnostic testing, when applicable, is often necessary to identify the causative trigger. Prompt recognition of anaphylaxis is prudent, and epinephrine is the first line for treatment. Despite the fact that epinephrine is always the recommended first line treatment for anaphylaxis, it is often underutilized in the clinical setting. Long-term management of anaphylaxis includes allergy referral, patient and caregiver education, access to epinephrine auto-injectors, and the development of an anaphylaxis or emergency care plan with regular review.

CLINICS CARE POINTS

- Anaphylaxis is a life-threatening systemic reaction caused by various mechanisms
- Patients experiencing anaphylaxis should be promptly treated with epinephrine as first-line management. Delaying treatment with epinephrine can lead to higher morbidity and mortality.

- After treatment for anaphylaxis, patients should be monitored until symptoms have fully resolved.
- Patients with the history of anaphylaxis should have an emergency care plan and access to an epinephrine auto-injector
- Patients with the history of anaphylaxis should be referred to allergy clinician and receive education on trigger avoidance, signs and symptoms of anaphylaxis, and proper use of epinephrine auto-injectors

DISCLOSURE

The authors have no commercial or financial conflicts of interest. No funding sources have been allotted for the publication of this article.

REFERENCES

1. Shaker MS, Wallac DV, Golden DBK, et al. Anaphylaxis-a 2020 practice parameter update, systematic review, and grading of recommendations, assessment, development and evaluation (GRADE) analysis. J Allergy Clin Immunol 2020; 145(4):1082–123.
2. Turner PJ, Worm M, Ansotegui IJ, et al. Time to revisit the definition and clinical criteria for anaphylaxis? World Allergy Organ J 2019;12(10):100066.
3. Lieberman P, Nicklas RA, Randolph C, et al. Anaphylaxis-a practice parameter update 2015. Ann Allergy Asthma Immunol 2015;115(5):341–84.
4. Sampson HA, Muñoz-Furlong A, Campbell RL, et al. Second symposium on the definition and management of anaphylaxis: summary report–Second National Institute of Allergy and Infectious Disease/Food Allergy and Anaphylaxis Network symposium. J Allergy Clin Immunol 2006;117(2):391–7.
5. Sampson HA, Aceves S, Bock SA, et al. Food allergy: a practice parameter update-2014. J Allergy Clin Immunol 2014;134(5):1016–25.
6. Sicherer SH, Muñoz-Furlong A, Godbold JH, et al. US prevalence of self-reported peanut, tree nut, and sesame allergy: 11-year follow-up. J Allergy Clin Immunol 2010;125(6):1322–6.
7. Nurmatov U, Dhami S, Arasi S, et al. Allergen immunotherapy for IgE-mediated food allergy: a systematic review and meta-analysis. Allergy 2017;72:1133–47.
8. Golden DBK, Moffitt J, Nickas RA, et al. Stinging insect hypersensitivity: a practice parameter update 2011. J Allergy Clin Immunol 2011;127(4):852–4.
9. Golden DBK, Demain J, Freeman T, et al. Stinging insect hypersensitivity: a practice parameter updated 2016. Ann Allergy Asthma Immunol 2017;118:28–54.
10. Joint Task Force on Practice Parameters. Drug allergy: an updated practice parameter. Ann Allergy Immunol 2010;105(4):259–73.
11. Parisi CAS, Kelly KJ, Ansotegui IJ, et al. Update on latex allergy: new insights into an old problem. World Allergy Organ J 2021;14:100569.
12. Cardona V, Ansotegui IJ, Ebisawa M, et al. World allergy organization anaphylaxis guidance 2020. World Allergy Organ J 2020;13:100472.

Asthma Chronic Obstructive Pulmonary Disease Overlap

Defining, Naming, Diagnosing, and Treating Asthma-Chronic Obstructive Pulmonary Disease Overlap

William D. Sanders, DMS, PA-C

KEYWORDS

- Asthma • COPD • ACO • Inflammation • Biomarkers • Eosinophils

KEY POINTS

- Patients with ACO are high utilizers of available medical resources.
- Debate over the name involves the Dutch verses British hypothesis.
- Clinical features of ACO relate to age, smoking history, history of atopy.
- Two inflammatory pathways (Th1 and Th2) are known.
- Some medications used for asthma, some for COPD, are effective for ACO.

INTRODUCTION

Physician assistants and other providers encounter patients with asthma and COPD on a regular basis. Most clinicians are familiar with these disease presentations and treat patients with each condition differently. Unresolved, however, is the approach they should use to treat patients who present with both conditions simultaneously.

Due to the inability to define it, asthma-COPD (chronic obstructive pulmonary disease) overlap (ACO) has been a topic of controversy since Orie's initial discussion of the overlap in 1961.[1] In 2014, personnel from the Global initiative for Chronic Obstructive Lung Disease and Global Initiative for Asthma (GOLD-GINA) published a document defining the asthma-COPD overlap syndrome (referred to as a syndrome at the time) "as characterized by persistent airflow limitation with several features usually associated with asthma and several features usually associated with COPD."[2] In 2020, GOLD published an update that indicated they would no longer use the term, ACO. Instead, they concluded that asthma and COPD are different disorders that

Allergy Specialty Care, 213 Southwest Main Boulevard, Lake City, FL 32025, USA
E-mail address: wdsanders04@comcast.net

Physician Assist Clin 8 (2023) 739–747
https://doi.org/10.1016/j.cpha.2023.06.003
2405-7991/23/© 2023 Elsevier Inc. All rights reserved.
physicianassistant.theclinics.com

could share common traits and clinical features such as eosinophilia and some degree of reversibility.[3]

Before scientific techniques such as genomics for pinpointing genes, gene expression, lipid and protein profiles, and the microbiome were available, Orie articulated what became known as the Dutch hypothesis; that asthma and COPD stemmed from a single disease. In other words, factors such as genetics and the environment influenced the clinical phenotype. Orie and colleagues phenotyped their patients; a process other researchers have since adopted.[1] The Dutch hypothesis positioned ACO in the middle of a spectrum that has asthma and COPD on opposite ends.

In contrast with the Dutch hypothesis, Fletcher proposed the British hypothesis in 1965 when he described the overlap as "a disease in which asthma and COPD occur as a result of different mechanisms triggered by different pathogeneses."[4] Under the British hypothesis, ACO has a *distinct and separate* pathogenesis from asthma and COPD.[5]

Gibson and Simpson (2009)[6] wrote that the 2007 Canadian guidelines for COPD indicated that clinicians were justified if they introduced inhaled corticosteroids for patients who had COPD with an asthma component. A couple of years later, Gibson and Simpson reintroduced the condition as an overlap of asthma and COPD. In 2017, GINA formally recommended the term, ACO, over the term "asthma COPD overlap syndrome" (ACOS) having decided the phenomena did not meet the definition of a syndrome.[7] Since the GINA-GOLD document published in 2014, interest and research in ACO has continued to increase. The articles covering the subject in PubMed alone had increased to more than 870 publications by April 2022.[8] Despite the growing interest, at the time of this writing, there was no universally accepted definition, and the GOLD update no longer referred to ACO. The most recent GINA update refers to Asthma-COPD overlap or asthma plus COPD, not as a definition but rather, as a descriptive term for clinical use that includes several different clinical phenotypes related to underlying mechanisms.[9]

LITERATURE REVIEW
Prevalence/incidence

Due to the absence of a precise definition and an increase in the heterogeneity of study populations, researchers have had difficulty in assessing the extent to which ACO has been prevalent in the U.S. population. According to Maselli and colleagues (2019),[10] ACO could exist in up to 27% of asthma and 33% of patients with COPD. Accurately defining asthma and other obstructive diseases is important for many reasons including improving the ability to determine prevalence, managing direct healthcare costs, and establishing guidelines. Patients with ACO were high utilizers of available medical resources, primarily because they were hospitalized more than patients with COPD or asthma alone, and hospitalizations have accounted for the largest proportion of healthcare costs for patients with COPD.[11] Additionally, researchers have found that patients with ACO have significantly worse prognoses and increased rates of mortality compared to patients with asthma and COPD alone.[12]

Clinical features

Clinicians can describe the differences between asthma and COPD by the unique characteristics of the two diseases. Asthma, for example, tends to start in childhood and is often related to allergies. Characteristic reversible airway obstructions usually lead to favorable prognoses. By contrast, COPD typically occurs in people over 40, is mostly related to tobacco smoking, and manifests as an airflow obstruction leading to a progressive decline in lung function and premature death.[13] These two diseases can have similar or overlapping features. Reddel and colleagues (2021)[14] found that a cross-sectional analysis of patients with a diagnosis of asthma and/or COPD, had marked heterogeneity within, and overlap between, each diagnostic label.

Obtaining meaningful data has been difficult because most clinical trials for asthma have excluded patients with features of COPD, and clinical trials for COPD have excluded patients with features of asthma. Notwithstanding, the data some researchers have acquired by studying discrete patient groups have been helpful. These patients with characteristics of asthma and COPD have included asthma patients who smoked and nonsmokers who developed COPD. Smoking asthmatics can have features similar to those with COPD. They tend to have more neutrophilic inflammation as compared to eosinophilia and are less responsive to corticosteroids.[6] Patients with COPD who received a diagnosis of asthma before the age of 40 often have: (1) more reversibility than patients with COPD alone, as seen on post-bronchodilator spirometry (change in forced expiratory ventilation in one second (FEV1) >12%, >200 mL); (2) peripheral eosinophilia; and (3) higher total immunoglobulin E (IgE).[15]

Protocols/criteria

Even if practitioners cannot agree on a precise definition, developing protocols for the diagnosis of ACO is useful because guidelines can lead to more effective treatment. For example, if a clinician diagnoses a patient with asthma as having ACO, adding an inhaler such as a long-acting beta2 agonist (LABA) or long-acting muscarinic antagonist (LAMA) can be a better strategy than prescribing high-dose oral corticosteroids, because clinicians can obtain comparable results without the side effects common with oral steroids. Correspondingly, when treating a COPD patient who has received a diagnosis of overlap, adding an inhaled corticosteroid to the treatment plan can improve that patient's lung function and clinical response.[16]

A global panel of experts, comprised of various specialists, from North America, Western Europe, and Asia met in 2016 and developed a consensus report on ACO. The panel decided on major and minor clinical, spirometric, and laboratory criteria. The major criteria included: (1) persistent airflow limitation in individuals 40 years old or older; (2) at least 10 pack-years of tobacco smoking *or* equivalent indoor or outdoor air pollution exposure; and (3) documented history of asthma before 40 years of age *or* producing a bronchodilator response (BDR) of > 400 mL in FEV1. The minor criteria included: (1) documented history of atopy or allergic rhinitis; (2) BDR of FEV1 $\geq$ 200 mL and 12% improvement from baseline values on two or more visits; and (3) peripheral blood eosinophil count of $\geq$ 300 cells/μL.[17] The authors felt this definition was more objective thus, when applied, facilitated diagnosis in daily clinical practice, since it included measures such as airway reversibility and peripheral blood eosinophil counts. Mekov and colleagues recommended that clinicians should consider patients who met all three major criteria and at least one minor criterion, for the diagnosis of ACO.

Pathogenesis and biomarkers

Three clinical features found in obstructive pulmonary diseases are airway inflammation, bronchial hyperresponsiveness, and airway obstruction. Scientists have thought chronic airway inflammation to be primarily eosinophilic in asthma driven by CD4 cells and neutrophilic in COPD driven by CD8 cells.[13] Asthma, as Fujino and Sugiur (2021)[18] explained, is a heterogenous disease resulting from an innate and adaptive inflammatory response leading to abnormal tissue remodeling and interleukins (IL)-4, IL-5, and IL-13. Those interleukins stimulate airway eosinophilia, mucus hypersecretion, bronchial hyperresponsiveness, and mast cell activation. Some scientists have suggested that inflammation originates from two different pathways. Inflammation in COPD is mostly mediated by T-helper 1(Th1) cells, and asthma is mediated by T-helper 2 (Th2) cells. Th1 cells produce interferon, interleukin −2, and tumor necrosis factor. Th2 produces several other interleukins (4,5,6,9,10, and 13). This causes a strong antibody response and eosinophil accumulation. Scientists, and clinicians alike, have referenced the inflammatory pathway activated by Th2 as *Type 2 inflammation*. Since COPD and asthma are heterogeneous diseases, these two inflammatory pathways can overlap in some patients causing a mixed pattern.[17] Data from administrative pharmacy and health care utilization have shown that high blood eosinophil counts were an independent risk factor for future exacerbations of COPD.[19]

Researchers have looked at type 2 inflammatory biomarkers such as fractionized expiratory nitric oxide (FeNO), blood eosinophils, and immunoglobulin E (IgE), to help distinguish ACO from asthma and COPD. There is a phenotype of patients with COPD who produce type 2 inflammatory cytokines that could manifest the clinical features of asthma (bronchodilator reversibility, increased peripheral eosinophilia). Researchers described these patients as having ACO.[20] In a study by Hiles, Gibson, and McDonald (2021),[21] researchers found that eosinophilic inflammation was common in patients with severe asthma, COPD, and ACO, but patients with ACO had more exacerbations requiring oral corticosteroids. The prevalence of eosinophilia was highest in patients who had ACO.[21]

Elevated FeNO and blood eosinophils typically correlate with local and systemic eosinophilic inflammation which is common with asthma. Markers of atopy, such as elevated total serum IgE and allergen-specific IgE levels, are also consistent with asthma, and clinicians have used these inflammatory biomarkers to support a diagnosis of ACO in patients with COPD.[22]

Two other markers of type 2 inflammation are serum periostin, a secreted extracellular matrix protein, and chitinase-3-like protein 1 (known as YKL-40). Researchers found periostin to be comparable in patients with asthma and ACO but lower in patients with COPD. YKL-40 is a secreted glycoprotein produced in macrophages, neutrophils, airway epithelium, and various cell types. Shirai and colleagues (2018)[23] found YKL-40 to be higher in COPD and ACO but not in asthma. Shirai and colleagues concluded that YKL-40, used together with serum periostin, could help in distinguishing ACO from asthma and COPD.

Ogata and colleagues (2022)[24] found that a transfer coefficient of the lung for carbon monoxide (KCO), similar, but superior, to the diffusing capacity of the lung for carbon monoxide (DLCO), was an independent risk factor for ACO. In the study, Ogata and colleagues (2022) reported that 30.9% of patients with ACO had low DLCO which was associated with decreased FEV1. Low DLCO is associated with alveolar destruction, namely emphysema, and is a prognostic marker for severe acute exacerbation in COPD.[25] Peng and colleagues (2022)[26] found that even adults who smoked with normal DLCO were more likely to be asthmatic.

Urine L-histidine and serum club cell secretory protein 16 (CC-16) could also be useful biomarkers.[27] As a result of studying a small prospective cohort of patients with chronic airway disease, Ogata and colleagues (2022)[24] found that, after adjusting for age, sex, and smoking amount, urinary L-histidine levels were higher in patients with ACO than in patients who had asthma or COPD alone. In this same sample of patients, ≥19 years of age and in a stable state for >3 months, CC-16 levels were lower in those who had ACO than in those who had asthma or COPD alone. CC-16 is one of the many club cell proteins that have a protective role in the respiratory system. These cells repair the airways after injury from harmful substances by secreting anti-inflammatory and immunomodulatory proteins.[28]

Therapeutic options

Treatment of ACO has been dependent on information extrapolated from asthma and COPD studies and on expert opinion rather than on evidence-based clinical trials.[12] Researchers found that patients with COPD with clinical features of asthma (particularly an elevated eosinophil count) had an increased FEV1 response when treated with inhaled corticosteroids (ICS)[29] These medications can be beneficial, nevertheless most clinicians have known that ICS can increase the risk of pneumonia in patients with COPD.[30]

As of this writing, authors of the GINA guidelines recommended that clinicians treat ACO-like asthma. Ishiura and colleagues (2019)[31] conducted a pilot study of 17 Japanese male patients with ACO, age range of 54-87 years to determine if combining inhaled medication (commonly used for asthma) with inhaled medication (commonly used for COPD) would be effective treatment for ACO. These commonly used medications included Umeclidinium (UMEC), a long-acting muscarinic antagonist indicated for COPD; Fluticasone furoate (FF), an inhaled corticosteroid; and vilanterol (VI), an inhaled long-acting bronchodilator combined in a single inhaler device, indicated for asthma and COPD. All participants were ex-smokers with a smoking history of 66.6 ± 39.5 pack-years ($\pm$SD). Ishiura and colleagues showed that lung function was improved from an FEV1 of 1.26 L, after the run-in period, to 1.33 L, after the FF/VI treatment period, and to 1.46 L after the UMEC plus FF/VI treatment period (the so-called triple therapy) which is the three medications (UMEC/FF/VI) in one inhaler.

Another potential treatment for ACO is the relatively new, targeted therapies known as biologics. The FDA in 2003 approved Omalizumab, a recombinant DNA-derived humanized monoclonal murine antibody[32] as the first biologic approved for asthma. Omalizumab, under the trade name Xolair, is an injection given every four weeks and targets free IgE, thus downregulating the sensitization of the immune system by preventing chronic activation of the Th2 responses.[33]

In March 2022, researchers at GINA[9] published the results of a multicenter, observational study with retrospective and prospective data collection to compare the responses of biologics used in patients with asthma and ACO. The researchers classified the patients into smokers (current or past smokers with a history of ≥ 10 pack-years) and nonsmokers and diagnosed smokers who showed bronchial obstruction (FEV1/FVC <70%). This followed GINA's proposal of smoking history, asthma features, and persistent expiratory airflow limitation with or without bronchodilator reversibility.[9] To assess clinical outcomes, researchers used the Asthma Control Test (ACT), severe exacerbations (hospital admission, emergency room visits, or the need for oral steroids for ≥ 3 days), unscheduled medical visits, the need for systemic corticosteroids, and the number of steroid bursts, all in the preceding 12 months. The authors defined clinical control as the absence of severe exacerbations in the previous year, ACT score of ≥ 20, and nonuse of systemic corticosteroids. Researchers included 24 patients diagnosed with ACO and 297 with asthma. They found FEV1 to be significantly lower ($p \leq .05$) in patients with ACO than those with asthma. However, the researchers found the biomarkers for type 2 inflammation similar in both groups as were the proportion of patients with atopy, chronic rhinosinusitis, and nasal polyps. Researchers found no significant difference in ACT scores after 12 months of biologic therapy between the two groups. Researchers did find the outcome variables showed better results for asthmatics, although 16% of the patients with ACO did achieve control from treatment with one of the biologic medications.[34]

DISCUSSION

Multiple researchers have found that patients with ACO are high utilizers of the health-care system[17,21,35] That underscores the need to identify these patients so clinicians can appropriately manage their illness with effective treatment. At the time of this article, there was no consensus over what to call patients who had both asthma and COPD, but interest in ACO and an increasing number of articles published provided evidence of their sustained interest. Since the GINA-GOLD document published in 2014, articles covering the subject in PubMed alone had increased to more than 870 publications by April 15, 2022.[8] This review emphasized the need to consider criteria such as smoking history, allergy history, age, BDR, FeNO, IgE, and other biomarkers so practitioners can make more accurate diagnoses and prescribe appropriate treatments. As of this writing, clinicians were utilizing treatments for ACO that they had previously used for asthma or COPD alone.

Pulmonologists, allergists, and other respiratory specialists have established major and minor criteria to help clinicians differentiate ACO from asthma and COPD. These criteria include age, smoking history, allergic history, and biomarkers. Spirometry is an objective biomarker, so clinicians should be able to apply these measurements in their clinical practice. Finding meaningful criteria is the first step in making a diagnosis and isolating these individuals so that they can receive appropriate treatment and management.

This researcher did not find a specific test pathognomonic for ACO in the literature, however, the literature lists many important biomarkers that can help clinicians diagnose ACO in patients. **Table 1** lists biomarkers used to distinguish asthma, COPD, and ACO. Clinicians have used Th2 biomarkers, such as blood eosinophils, FeNO, and IgE (that are helpful in categorizing asthma phenotypes), to distinguish ACO from COPD.

Researchers found serum periostin and YKL-40, two other biomarkers of type two inflammation, to be useful in distinguishing ACO from asthma and COPD when used together. KCO and DLCO are biomarkers clinicians can use to predict exacerbations in ACO. Additionally, Urine L-histidine and CC-16 may be effective biomarkers to separate ACO from asthma and COPD, but further research is needed.

Treating patients who have ACO can be confusing for clinicians because there is no consensual agreement on how to identify the condition. The literature did, however, provide some insight on how to direct therapy. The so-called "triple therapy" which includes a long-acting bronchodilator, a long-acting muscarinic antagonist, and an inhaled corticosteroid, showed improved lung function in patients with ACO. In addition to inhalers that broncho-dilate and those that reduce inflammation

Table 1
Biomarkers for asthma, COPD, and ACO

Biomarkers	Asthma	COPD	ACO
Blood eosinophils	Commonly increased	Dec	Often increased
FeNO	Commonly increased	Dec	Often increased
IgE	Often increased	Dec	Often increased
Periostin	Equal to ACO pts	Dec	Equal to asthma pts
YKL-40	Not increased	Inc	Increased
KCO/DLCO	Normal	Low	Low in 1/3 pts
Urine L-histidine			Higher than asthma and COPD alone
CC-16			Lower than asthma and COPD alone

(corticosteroids), the new "biologics" class of medicines target specific mediators of inflammation and showed improvement in lung function and symptoms of patients with asthma. One of the biologics (omalizumab), showed improvement in patients with ACO. Research of other biologics was ongoing when this researcher conducted this study.

Researchers and clinicians alike have become more knowledgeable about the pathophysiology of asthma, COPD, and ACO since Orie first discussed the combination in 1961. All three conditions are heterogeneous and involve a cascade of events consisting of genetic, innate, and adaptive immune responses. These responses, for COPD and asthma, are manifested as inflammation and are mediated (mostly) by Th1 and Th2 cells, respectively. These two pathways produce their own inflammatory mediators including a variety of interleukins, interferon, and tumor necrosis factor. Th2 (type 2 inflammation) promotes a strong antibody response, driving eosinophils to the area causing accumulation. The heterogeneity of COPD and asthma is such that the Th1 and Th2 pathways can overlap in some cases which leads to a mixed pattern as seen in ACO.

Regardless of whether ACO is a separate disease or exists on a spectrum between asthma and COPD, it is a real phenomenon that deserves a diagnosis that differs from that used for asthma and COPD. With continued interest and ongoing studies, researchers are likely to find diagnostic biomarkers that will lead to the discovery of novel treatments. The hope is that these discoveries can lead to the development of an effective framework of diagnosis and treatment that frontline clinicians can easily apply. When this happens, medical providers will be able to effectively manage this special group of patients, leading to lower hospital admission rates and reduced healthcare burden.

CLINICS CARE POINTS

- When evaluating a patient with asthma, details in the history (10 pack-years of tobacco smoking, post-bronchodilator non-reversibility) can lead to a diagnosis of ACO.
- When evaluating a patient with COPD, look for clues such as a history of atopy, asthma before age 40, elevated FeNO, eosinophils, and post-bronchodilator response to diagnose ACO.
- Periostin, YKL-40, KCO, Urine L-histidine, and CC-16 are potentially useful biomarkers but may not be available in many practice areas.
- If deciding on treatment for patients with ACO, consider "triple therapy" which includes a long-acting bronchodilator, a long-acting muscarinic antagonist, and an inhaled corticosteroid.
- If not controlled on inhalers, consider biologic medications to target specific mediators of inflammation.

DISCLOSURE

The author has nothing to disclose.

REFERENCES

1. Postma DS, Weiss ST, van den Berge M, et al. Revisiting the dutch hypothesis. J Allergy Clin Immunol 2015;136(3):521–9.

2. 2014_Diagnosis of diseases of chronic airflow limitation.pdf. pg4. Available at: https://ginasthma.org/wp-content/uploads/2019/11/GINA_GOLD_ACOS_2014-wms.pdf. Accessed October 26, 2021.

3. Roman-Rodriguez M, Kaplan A. GOLD 2021 strategy report: implications for asthma–COPD overlap. Int J Chronic Obstr Pulm Dis 2021;16:1709–15.

4. Hikichi M, Hashimoto S, Gon Y. Asthma and COPD overlap pathophysiology of ACO. Allergol Int 2018;67(2):179–86.

5. Albertson TE, Chenoweth JA, Pearson SJ, et al. The pharmacological management of asthma-chronic obstructive pulmonary disease overlap syndrome (ACOS). Expet Opin Pharmacother 2020;21(2):213–31.

6. Gibson PG, Simpson JL. The overlap syndrome of asthma and COPD: what are its features and how important is it? Thorax 2009;64(8):728–35.

7. Yanagisawa S, Ichinose M. Definition and diagnosis of asthma–COPD overlap (ACO). Allergol Int 2018;67(2):172–8.

8. Fouka E, Papaioannou AI, Hillas G, et al. Asthma-COPD overlap syndrome: recent insights and unanswered questions. J Personalized Med 2022;12(5):708.

9. Global Initiative for Asthma. Global Strategy for Asthma Management and Prevention. Global Initiative for Asthma; 2022. Available at: https://ginasthma.org/wp-content/uploads/2022/07/GINA-Main-Report-2022-FINAL-22-07-01-WMS.pdf. Accessed November 6, 2022.

10. Maselli DJ, Hardin M, Christenson SA, et al. Clinical Approach to the Therapy of Asthma-COPD Overlap. Chest 2019;155(1):168–77.

11. Tho NV, Park HY, Nakano Y. Asthma-COPD overlap syndrome (ACOS): a diagnostic challenge. Respirology 2016;21(3):410–8.

12. Hahn DL. Does the asthma-chronic obstructive pulmonary disease overlap syndrome (ACOS) exist? A narrative review from epidemiology and practice. Allergol Immunopathol 2022;50(6):100–6.

13. Papaiwannou A, Zarogoulidis P, Porpodis K, et al. Asthma-chronic obstructive pulmonary disease overlap syndrome (ACOS): current literature review. J Thorac Dis 2014;6(Suppl 1):S146–51.

14. Reddel HK, Vestbo J, Agustí A, et al. Heterogeneity within and between physician-diagnosed asthma and/or COPD: NOVELTY cohort. Eur Respir J 2021;58(3). https://doi.org/10.1183/13993003.03927-2020.

15. Barrecheguren M, Román-Rodríguez M, Miravitlles M. Is a previous diagnosis of asthma a reliable criterion for asthma–COPD overlap syndrome in a patient with COPD? Int J Chronic Obstr Pulm Dis 2015;10:1745–52.

16. Shabaan AY, Daabis RG, Abdelhady AM, et al. Prevalence of asthma—chronic obstructive pulmonary disease overlap in patients with airflow limitation. The Egyptian Journal of Bronchology 2021;15(1):4.

17. Mekov E, Nuñez A, Sin DD, et al. Update on asthma–COPD overlap (ACO): a narrative review. COPD 2021;16:1783–99.

18. Fujino N, Sugiura H. ACO (Asthma–COPD Overlap) is independent from copd, a case in favor: a systematic review. Diagnostics 2021;11(5):859.

19. Zeiger RS, Tran TN, Butler RK, et al. Relationship of blood eosinophil count to exacerbations in chronic obstructive pulmonary disease. J Allergy Clin Immunol Pract 2018;6(3):944–54.e5.

20. Khanduja D, Kajal NC, Mathew L, et al. A case study on asthma-COPD Overlap (ACO) is independent from COPD. Archives of Pulmonology and Respiratory Care 2021;7(1):020.

21. Hiles SA, Gibson PG, McDonald VM. Disease burden of eosinophilic airway disease: comparing severe asthma, COPD and asthma–COPD overlap. Respirology 2021;26(1):52–61.
22. Kobayashi S, Hanagama M, Yamanda S, et al. Inflammatory biomarkers in asthma-COPD overlap syndrome. Int J Chronic Obstr Pulm Dis 2016;11:2117–23.
23. Shirai T, Hirai K, Gon Y, et al. Combined assessment of serum periostin and YKL-40 may identify asthma-COPD overlap. J Allergy Clin Immunol Pract 2018;7. https://doi.org/10.1016/j.jaip.2018.06.015.
24. Ogata H, Katahira K, Enokizu-Ogawa A, et al. The association between transfer coefficient of the lung and the risk of exacerbation in asthma-COPD overlap: an observational cohort study. BMC Pulm Med 2022;22(1):22.
25. Choi J, Sim JK, Oh JY, et al. Prognostic marker for severe acute exacerbation of chronic obstructive pulmonary disease: analysis of diffusing capacity of the lung for carbon monoxide (DLCO) and forced expiratory volume in one second (FEV1). BMC Pulm Med 2021;21(1):152.
26. Peng J, Wang M, Wu Y, et al. Clinical indicators for asthma-COPD overlap: a systematic review and meta-analysis. Int J Chronic Obstr Pulm Dis 2022;17:2567–75.
27. Jo YS. Status of studies investigating asthma–chronic obstructive pulmonary disease overlap in korea: a review. Tuberc Respir Dis 2022;85(2):101–10.
28. Oh JY, Lee YS, Min KH, et al. Decreased serum club cell secretory protein in asthma and chronic obstructive pulmonary disease overlap: a pilot study. Int J Chronic Obstr Pulm Dis 2018;13:3411–7.
29. Kitaguchi Y, Komatsu Y, Fujimoto K, et al. Sputum eosinophilia can predict responsiveness to inhaled corticosteroid treatment in patients with overlap syndrome of COPD and asthma. Int J Chronic Obstr Pulm Dis 2012;7:283–9.
30. Anigati E, Verma S, Khanijo S. Asthma–chronic obstructive pulmonary disease overlap syndrome – a brief review. Egypt J Chest Dis Tuberc 2022;71(2):139.
31. Ishiura Y, Fujimura M, Ohkura N, et al. Effect of triple therapy in patients with asthma-COPD overlap. Int J Clin Pharmacol Ther 2019;57(8):384–92.
32. Louie S, Zeki AA, Schivo M, et al. The asthma–chronic obstructive pulmonary disease overlap syndrome: pharmacotherapeutic considerations. Expet Rev Clin Pharmacol 2013;6(2):197–219.
33. Kusumoto M, Mathis BJ. Biologic treatments for asthma and chronic obstructive pulmonary disorder. Allergie 2021;1(2):92–107.
34. Pérez de Llano L, Dacal Rivas D, Marina Malanda N, et al. The response to biologics is better in patients with severe asthma than in patients with asthma–copd overlap syndrome. J Asthma Allergy 2022;15:363–9.
35. Mendy A, Forno E, Niyonsenga T, et al. Prevalence and features of asthma-COPD overlap in the U.S. 2007-2012. Clin Respir J 2018;12(8):2369–77.

Moving?

Make sure your subscription moves with you!

To notify us of your new address, find your **Clinics Account Number** (located on your mailing label above your name), and contact customer service at:

Email: journalscustomerservice-usa@elsevier.com

800-654-2452 (subscribers in the U.S. & Canada)
314-447-8871 (subscribers outside of the U.S. & Canada)

Fax number: 314-447-8029

Elsevier Health Sciences Division
Subscription Customer Service
3251 Riverport Lane
Maryland Heights, MO 63043

*To ensure uninterrupted delivery of your subscription, please notify us at least 4 weeks in advance of move.

Printed and bound by CPI Group (UK) Ltd, Croydon, CR0 4YY

03/10/2024

01040476-0012